S0-BQH-687

THINGS YOU OUGHT TO KNOW ABOUT
YOUR CHANGING BODY AND YOURSELF:

Are heart attacks as dangerous as you fear?
How common is excess sugar in the blood?
Are you ever too old for sex?
What is at the root of gastric discomfort?
Can loss of vision or hearing be averted if caught in time?
How safe is aspirin?
What does it mean if you are short-winded?
Do high-fiber diets live up to their claims?

These are just a few of the questions answered
fully, fairly, and understandably in—

THE DOCTORS' GUIDE TO GROWING OLDER

SANDOR A. FRIEDMAN is Professor of Medicine at the State University of New York Downstate Medical Center. He is chief of the Peripheral Vascular Disease Division of Coney Island Hospital, where he also holds the post of Chief of Medical Services. Dr. Friedman is a Fellow of the American Geriatric Society.

FRANCIS U. STEINHEBER is an Assistant Professor of Clinical Medicine at New York University School of Medicine. He is Chief of Gastroenterology at Coney Island Hospital and a Fellow of the American College of Physicians.

ABRAHAM H. LASS, an educator with over forty years of experience, is presently educational consultant to Coney Island Hospital. He is a member of the American Medical Writers Association.

THE DOCTORS' GUIDE TO
GROWING OLDER

Sandor A. Friedman. M.D.
Francis U. Steinheber. M.D.
Abraham H. Lass

Illustrations by Charles Stern

A PLUME BOOK
NEW AMERICAN LIBRARY
TIMES MIRROR
NEW YORK, LONDON AND SCARBOROUGH, ONTARIO

*We dedicate this book to our patients and students,
from whom we continue to learn.*

Publisher's Note
The ideas, procedures, and suggestions contained in this book
are not intended as a substitute for consulting with
your physician. All matters regarding your health
require medical supervision.

Copyright © 1980 by Sandor A. Friedman, Francis U. Steinheber,
and Abraham H. Lass

Illustrations copyright © 1980 by The New American Library, Inc.

All rights reserved

SIGNET, SIGNET CLASSICS, MENTOR, PLUME, MERIDIAN and
NAL BOOKS are published *in the United States* by The New
American Library, Inc., 1633 Broadway, New York, New York 10019,
in Canada by The New American Library of Canada Limited,
81 Mack Avenue, Scarborough, Ontario M1L 1M8,
in the United Kingdom by The New English Library Limited,
Barnard's Inn, Holborn, London EC1N 2JR, England

First Printing, October, 1980

1   2   3   4   5   6   7   8   9

PRINTED IN THE UNITED STATES OF AMERICA

ACKNOWLEDGMENTS

The authors wish to thank Dr. Judith Friedman, who contributed the chapter "Sex—Good at Any Age." We also wish to thank the following physicians for their helpful suggestions:

Dr. Harry Bienenstock
Chief, Division of Rheumatology
Coney Island Hospital
Clinical Assistant Professor of Medicine
Cornell University School of Medicine

Dr. Santi Dhar
Chief, Division of Pulmonary Disease
Coney Island Hospital
Assistant Professor of Medicine
State University of New York
Downstate Medical Center

Dr. Chai Dharapak
Chief, Department of Orthopedics
Coney Island Hospital

Dr. Leslie Fine
Chief, Department of Psychiatry
Coney Island Hospital

Dr. Ernst Greif
Chief, Division of Cardiology
Coney Island Hospital
Assistant Professor of Medicine
State University of New York
Downstate Medical Center

Dr. Emily Karp
Chief, Ophthalmology Department
Coney Island Hospital
Assistant Professor Department of Surgery
State University of New York
Downstate Medical Center

Dr. Norman Posner
Director, Department of Obstetrics & Gynecology
Associate Professor of Obstetrics & Gynecology
State University of New York
Downstate Medical Center

Dr. Herman Rosen
Chief, Nephrology Division
Coney Island Hospital
Associate Professor of Clinical Medicine
State University of New York
Downstate Medical Center

Dr. Stanley Wein
Chief, Division of Otolaryngology
Coney Island Hospital
Associate Attending Physician
Maimonides Medical Center

Dr. Mary Wheeler
Chief, Division of Endocrinology & Metabolism
Coney Island Hospital
Assistant Professor of Medicine
State University of New York
Downstate Medical Center

Finally, we are indebted to our indefatigable secretary,
Ms. Edna Flug, who typed many drafts of this manuscript
efficiently and accurately.

CONTENTS

vii

FOREWORD

This book represents the combined efforts of two physicians (Sandor A. Friedman and Francis U. Steinheber) and a professional educator (Abraham H. Lass) who came to know each other under unique circumstances. One of us (AHL) is a retired high school principal who wanted to continue his long-term commitment to education. In 1974, he came to Coney Island Hospital, a busy municipal institution in New York City, to offer his services in the educational program for the young doctors in training.

It was here that we first met and began to develop the close and continuing personal and professional relationships that made this book possible.

Almost immediately we were caught up in discussions of the kind of medical care most people should and actually do receive. We were soon deep into what we considered a central, crucial problem in doctor-patient relationships: the failure of doctors to communicate fully and effectively with their patients—and, of course, the inevitable failure of patients to understand fully what their doctors were trying to tell them.

Friedman and Steinheber wondered why so many of their patients understood very little about the illnesses they had lived with for years. Speaking as a patient with a varied exposure to different kinds of doctors, Lass suggested that faulty communication, in large measure, starts with the doctors themselves. They just do not tell their patients enough about what ails them. This is not true of all doctors, of course, but of a sufficiently large number to give considerable credence to this generalization.

There are some good reasons for patients' widely felt and expressed complaint: "My doctor doesn't talk to me. My doctor doesn't tell me anything." Some doctors are too busy —or *think* they are too busy to tell their patients what they should know about themselves and their illnesses. Others are just not very good communicators. They have mastered their medicine. They are zealous in getting at their patients' difficulties and in applying the best that today's medical science has to offer. But nowhere in their medical school and hospital preparation have they learned or been taught the immensely difficult and subtle art of talking to their patients. In addition, many doctors feel (and probably rightly so) that their patients do not know enough basic facts about how their bodies work. Giving these people even what the doctor thinks is a simple explanation raises the very real possibility of compounding their confusion and creating even more problems for doctor and patient. So, some doctors have reluctantly concluded, the less they tell their patients the better.

Patients are not wholly without blame for this communication gap between their doctors and themselves. Some don't really listen to what their doctors tell them: they hear only a part of what they are being told—and frequently remember only part of what they hear. Others are intimidated by their doctors and are ashamed to ask for understandable explanations of their illnesses and the effects of prescribed medication.

So we pooled the insights and experiences of our three lifetimes and wrote this book in an effort to bridge the communication gap between doctor and patient.

This book is about the awesome, incredibly complex, and delicately put-together human body—and what happens to it in time. It deals with the medical problems that come upon us as we grow older. Obviously none of us will have all of these problems. And none of us will escape them entirely. In one form or another, at one time or another, we shall encounter our fair share of them.

What can you do about these problems? Several things. Realize that a great many are treatable, curable, tolerable. You can, like hundreds of thousands, lead a pleasant, useful life with many of these problems. And you can, as this book will show you, avoid some of them.

Understand yourself and your problems.

Giving you this understanding has been one of our major concerns in writing this book. That is why we have taken such pains to explain in detail, in simple language and graphic sketches, the various conditions you and your friends and relatives may have.

We believe very strongly that you have the right to know what's wrong with you—precisely, specifically, physically, emotionally. So, for example, if you should have hypertension or diabetes, a careful reading of these sections in this book will give you more than a name or label for what's ailing you. You'll find out what is happening inside you and what medications will and won't do to help you.

Do something to help yourself.

1. Recognize the early signs of trouble. You'll find this book will help you.
2. Get to your doctor as soon as possible.
3. Get proper treatment as soon as possible.
4. Know what to look for in your doctor and what questions to ask him about yourself (see Chapter 20, Choosing a Doctor).

The conditions we have dealt with in this book occur in almost every age group. Diabetes, for example, can be found among the very young. Hypertension is not exclusively an older person's problem. Nor is arthritis or stomach or heart trouble. It is true, however, that as we grow older we tend to be more intensely and more frequently affected by many of the ailments we have dealt with here.

So this book is designed to speak to the problems of

various kinds of people. First, those who by any reasonable standards are getting older. They aren't functioning the way they used to. Unpleasant, unexpected things are happening to them. They will learn from this book what may be causing their difficulties, what modern medicine can do for them, and what they can do for themselves to prevent further problems and to deal positively with those they now have.

We also address those who are on the way to getting older. This book will give them some notion about what may be in store for them in the years ahead—much of it preventable in some measure. We hope this will enable them to meet their futures with courage, equanimity, and even good humor.

And lastly, we are directing this book to those whose care and understanding we shall need sooner or later—our children, our relatives, our friends, our doctors, nurses, and other professionals.

We hope our readers will recognize in these pages our common needs and our common destiny.

S.A.F.
F.U.S.
August 1980   A.H.L.

THE DOCTORS'
GUIDE TO
GROWING
OLDER

1

HARDENING OF THE ARTERIES (ARTERIOSCLEROSIS) AND POOR CIRCULATION

At one time or another many people complain about "poor circulation." Their complaints and symptoms take various forms:

I feel tired, "rotten," under the weather.
I feel cold all the time.
My feet are cold, my hands are cold.
I wake up at night with cramps in my legs.
My toes and fingers tingle, feel numb, "fall asleep."

These are very real complaints and can be very worrisome. But they aren't all caused by what is popularly and inaccurately called *poor circulation*.

The best antidote for ignorance or insufficient knowledge is a proper dose of simple, accurate information and understanding. So we're going to devote this chapter to an explanation of what your circulation really is, how it works normally, and what happens to you when something goes wrong with it.

The circulation is really the freight system of the body. Just as freight trains and trucks carry farm and industrial products to outlets all over the country and return defective and unused merchandise to factories, our bloodstream fulfills a similar role. The engine of the circulation is the heart that pumps blood through arteries all over the body. These arteries deliver the energy sources (primarily sugar and oxygen) along with vital minerals, vitamins, and proteins. In this chapter, we shall be concentrating on the arteries and what can happen to them.

ARTERIES

Arteries are thick tubes or pipes that have two important characteristics: strength and elasticity. They are similar to a series of branches in a large tree. The trunk of this arterial tree is the main artery, called the *aorta*, which carries the blood from the heart into the branches. Each branch artery, such as those to the head, arms, legs, kidneys, and intestinal tract, diverges further into progressively smaller branches that cover every inch of the body. The very small branches are called *arterioles*.

The walls of the arteries contain their own muscles as well as long fibers called elastic tissue, which stretch and relax much like a rubber band. This elastic tissue keeps the circulation of blood flowing smoothly and continuously. If the arteries were just like iron pipes, blood would pump through the system while the heart was pumping, but there would be only a trickle dripping through the system between heartbeats. By stretching when the heart pumps blood against their walls, the arteries store energy. While the heart rests between beats, they snap back like a rubber band, and this force keeps the blood moving throughout the body.

This elasticity also protects the arteries from damage caused by the force of blood against their walls. The analogy to trees is again useful. In a hurricane, thick, heavy trees are more likely to fall than more delicate, flexible ones because the latter sway more easily. A stretching object diffuses the impact of a blow in contrast to a rigid object that absorbs the full force.

The arterioles (smallest arteries) have an additional

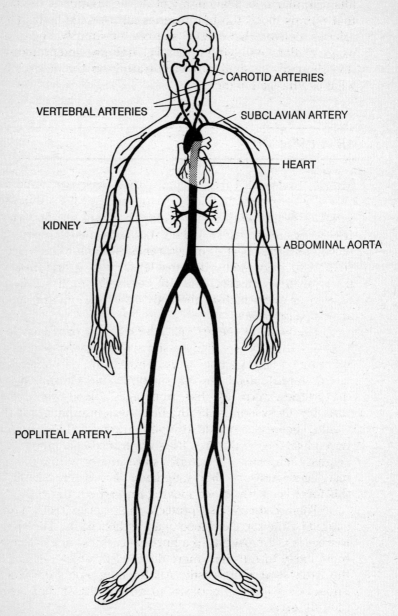

Fig. 1 Normal circulation.

characteristic. They are supplied with a great number of specialized nerve fibers called *sympathetic nerves*. When these nerves stimulate the muscles of arterioles, these muscles shorten (contract) just like the muscles in our arms and legs. The result is to narrow the arterioles so that less blood can go through them. When the nerves stop stimulating the arterioles, the muscles relax and the arterioles open again. This reversible closing and opening is called *vasoconstriction* and *vasodilatation*.

ARTERIOSCLEROSIS

This term is used to describe a number of changes that make arteries stiffer and clog their centers. Although arteriosclerosis is, in one sense, a disease, it is also a normal part of aging. Many studies have shown that changes in the arteries begin as early as childhood and progress gradually over a period of years. The arteries do not suddenly harden. It takes a long time before the symptoms of arteriosclerosis begin to appear.

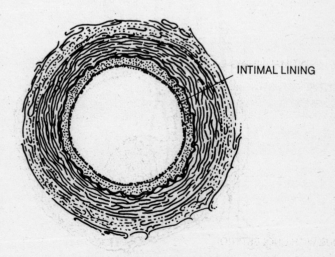

INTIMAL LINING

Fig. 2   Lining of normal artery.

Basically, two things happen to an artery undergoing arteriosclerosis. First, the lining of the artery (*intima*) is damaged by the accumulation of cholesterol, calcium, and other substances from the blood. These form in plaques called *atheromas*. The plaques continue to enlarge, develop jagged edges, and cause further damage to the artery's wall. Blood clots form on these plaques and lead to more damage. This vicious cycle continues until the entire arterial tube is closed off.

The other change involves loss of elasticity. The artery may become rigid and can no longer stretch like a rubber band. The two processes, loss of elasticity and injury to the lining, do not necessarily occur at the same time.

POOR CIRCULATION IN THE LEGS

For unknown reasons, the arteries in the arms rarely grow hard, but symptoms of arteriosclerosis are quite common in the legs of people over fifty. Men have these symptoms

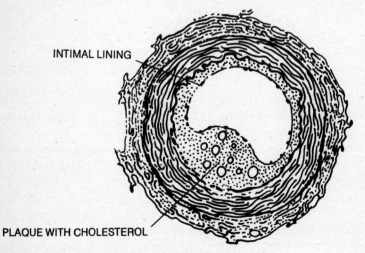

INTIMAL LINING

PLAQUE WITH CHOLESTEROL

Fig. 3   Lining of artery with arteriosclerosis.

much more often than women probably because their hormones are different. Female hormones seem to protect
women against arteriosclerosis. After the menopause and
particularly in the later decades, women tend to get the
same number of circulatory problems as men.

The most characteristic symptom of poor circulation in
the legs is called *intermittent claudication*. Claudication is a
very easily recognized kind of pain because it occurs only
when you walk. That is when the leg muscles do not receive
enough oxygen. It appears in only one of two areas—the
calf of the leg or around the buttocks and hips. The pain
varies greatly from person to person. For some, it may be
sharp and knifelike or just a cramp. Most people, however,
describe a tightening or squeezing sensation in their legs
that comes on suddenly and quickly becomes unbearable.

The symptoms of claudication occur when you are
walking. You always feel this pain if you walk far enough,
and the distance necessary for bringing it on remains fairly
constant from day to day under the same conditions. Cold
weather and fast walking will bring on the pain sooner. If
you have claudication, depending on how serious it is, you
will begin to experience pain after walking anywhere from
half a block to four or five blocks. The weather might affect
it by one block either way. The claudication symptoms always go away within a few minutes when you stop walking.
After the pain stops, you can generally walk a similar distance before pain starts again. So, even with claudication,
you can walk for miles as long as you rest each time the pain
occurs.

One strange feature of intermittent claudication is the
effect that the walking surface can have on your walking
ability. People who cannot walk more than two or three
blocks on an ordinary sidewalk without stopping can walk
much longer distances on a more springy surface such as a
boardwalk.

Most pains are not symptoms of claudication. Pain
around the joints and low-back pain aggravated by bending
are usually due to some form of arthritis and have nothing to
do with the circulation or claudication. Tired feelings in the
legs, which may occur quite often in people who are seden-

tary and out of shape, are not circulation problems. Nor are leg cramps developing at rest or in bed at night. These cramps are common, not serious, and they are relieved by walking. If they occur frequently, your doctor can give you bedtime medication to prevent them.

COLD FEET

Poor circulation may make your feet feel cold. Our blood is warm and thus warms our skin as it travels through the arteries in the skin. Naturally, a foot with clogged arteries will be colder than other parts of the body because it receives less blood. But this is only one of many reasons for cold feet. This coldness is usually the result of temporary narrowing of the small arteries (vasoconstriction) that we mentioned earlier in this chapter. This narrowing will occur if you are in a cold place or become anxious or emotionally upset. Some of us are prone to this under normal conditions. In fact, many normal, calm people have cold feet and hands a good deal of the time.

We must distinguish this normal feeling of coldness from coldness caused by circulatory problems. The foot with clogged arteries is cold all the time. There is nothing wrong with the circulation of the foot that is often cold when you first get into bed but is warm when you awaken in the morning. If only one foot is cold, it is likely that you do have a circulatory problem. If both feet are cold and you cannot remember when they were warm, you probably do not have a circulatory problem.

PINS AND NEEDLES

A feeling of pins and needles or numbness in the feet or toes is fairly common. Everyone has experienced this occasionally, especially after sitting in a cramped position for a long time. After a brief walk, the sensation wears off. If this numbness happens to you often and is associated with increasing coldness, you may have a circulatory problem, and a doctor should evaluate your symptom carefully.

There are many causes of numbness that have nothing to do with circulation. Very often, numbness means that the nerves of the feet have been damaged. A wide variety of diseases, including diabetes, kidney disease, alcoholism, and arthritis of the spine, can affect these nerves and produce numbness.

FOOT PAIN WHILE AT REST

This pain, when due to poor circulation, is characteristically severe and has a burning quality to it even though the foot is cold. It means that the foot is not receiving sufficient oxygen to meet its relatively small needs even when it is resting. This "rest pain" is a very serious symptom. If it is not treated promptly, the foot may become gangrenous. With gangrene, the cells of the foot actually turn black and die, and the foot must be amputated. Again, however, most foot pains have nothing to do with the circulation.

EXAMINATION AND TREATMENT OF LEGS WITH CIRCULATORY PROBLEMS

There are several clues that your physician will look for when he examines your legs. First, he will feel the pulses in your legs. The pulse of blood in the artery can normally be felt in the groin (femoral artery), in the back of the knee (popliteal artery), on the inside of the ankle (posterior tibial artery), and on top of the foot (dorsalis pedis artery). If one or more of the first three pulses is absent or weak, your doctor will know immediately that you have some blockage in your arteries. A missing dorsalis pedis pulse may be a normal finding in some people.

He will determine whether one foot is cooler than the other, and he will look carefully at the skin and its color. A pale foot or one that becomes blue when it is lowered has insufficient blood flow. If you see these color changes on your own, get to your doctor immediately.

Treatment of poor circulation in the legs depends on how serious the problem is. People with this problem fall into one of three categories:

1. Those with no symptoms

2. Those who have only intermittent claudication
3. Those who have pain in the foot at rest or important color changes in the foot.

The vast majority of people are in Group I. Although they have clogged arteries, their bodies have been able to open new arteries (collateral circulation) to offset most of the blockage. So they have a normal or nearly normal blood supply. Your doctor can determine that you have artery disease on routine examination if he notes the absence of one or more of the pulses. Treatment in this case really is preventive medicine. Your foot is receiving enough blood for normal conditions, but the blood supply may not be adequate for handling extraordinary conditions. For example, an open sore or infection might increase the need for blood beyond what can be delivered, and gangrene may ensue. We routinely give our patients with circulation problems a printed list of instructions concerning the care of their feet:

1. Tobacco: Do not smoke.
2. Cold: Avoid extreme cold. Dress very warmly in winter. Do not bathe or swim in cold water.
3. Heat: Never apply heat or ice to the feet. Avoid exposure of feet or legs to the sun.
4. Position: Sleep with your legs on the level with the bed. Never sit with your legs crossed.
5. Cleanliness: Wash your feet with a mild soap. Lukewarm water only. Dry feet carefully, especially between toes.
6. Dry, scaly skin: You may apply lanolin or cold cream to your feet. Gently massage into the dry, scaly areas.
7. Toenails: Should be cut by a podiatrist or a member of your family. Cut the toenails straight across and never cut in at the corners or too close to the skin.
8. Corns and calluses: Should be taken care of by a podiatrist.
9. Shoes and socks: Never walk in your bare feet. Wear only comfortable, properly fitting shoes and socks. Square or round-toed shoes are preferable.

Wear a clean pair of socks each day. Do not wear circular garters or hose with elastic tops.

10. Local medication: Never use strong antiseptics, tincture of iodine, corn remedies, or corn plasters on your feet. Use only medications ordered by your doctor.

11. Exercise: Walking is a good way to improve your circulation.

12. Injuries: Try to avoid even minor injuries to your feet by following the above rules. Consult your doctor at the first sign of discomfort in your legs or any injury to your legs or feet.

13. Self-inspection: You may not be able to feel pain in your feet as well as you should. Therefore, examine your feet every two or three days. If there are cracks or cuts in the skin or color changes, see your doctor even if you have no pain.

Two items on the above list require special emphasis. A foot with poor circulation is very sensitive to temperature extremes. Putting it in cold water will decrease its circulation. A hot bath or electric blanket may burn it. If you cannot feel temperature differences, you may place your feet in water that is too hot or too cold without realizing it. Therefore, *check bath and shower water with your elbows*.

Very few people with mild arterial blockage will ever have any serious problems with their feet if they follow these instructions carefully. On the other hand, you can run into a great deal of trouble and even lose a leg if you burn your foot in a hot bath, wear poorly fitting shoes, or cut your skin.

People with intermittent claudication require careful, individually tailored treatment. Many of these people are overweight and heavy smokers. If you have claudication, your doctor will urge you to lose weight, stop smoking, and walk as much as possible. You can walk for miles every day if you allow enough time for rest when the pain appears. There is an excellent chance that your condition may improve during the first four to six months. Exercise stimulates the opening of spare arteries, and you may be able to walk away your claudication.

The only medication available for treating intermittent claudication is a group of drugs called *vasodilators*. These drugs act directly on the arterial walls, relaxing their muscles and opening the channel a little bit. The pharmaceutical companies do a great deal of advertising to promote these medications, but a number of careful studies have failed to corroborate their claims. In normal walking, we must increase our blood flow to our leg muscles by 500 to 1000 percent. In contrast, these vasodilator drugs increase blood flow very little. It is our opinion that these drugs are not useful for treating intermittent claudication.

WHEN DO YOU NEED AN OPERATION?

If you do not improve with a conservative approach, your doctor must decide whether surgery is advisable. In an operation called *arterial bypass*, the surgeon attaches a plastic tube to a large artery on both sides of the clogged portion. Blood can then flow around the blocked area through this tube. This operation in selected cases is highly successful in restoring the circulation to normal.

There are several factors for your doctor to consider before recommending surgery. First, he must assess your general health and make sure that you can withstand a three-hour surgical procedure.

Second, your individual life-style counts for much. How important is it for you to be able to walk a longer distance without stopping? Does your occupation require you to do much continuous walking? Do you have to walk quickly? Do you like to take long walks? These are some of the questions that you must answer for yourself and your doctor.

Few jobs require continuous walking, and so claudication rarely interferes with one's employment. Most people can adjust their life-styles to a moderate amount of claudication without too much trouble.

If you and your doctor agree that you are fit for an arterial bypass operation, you must first be hospitalized for a special X-ray test called an *arteriogram*. In this test, a special dye is injected into the artery in the groin so that it can travel through the arterial system. By following the flow of the dye with a series of X-rays, the surgeon can see the area of blockage. From these pictures, he can determine whether it is technically possible to do the operation. In general, the operation is possible only in the larger arteries. The arteriogram test should not be performed unless you have already decided that you want surgery. Although the test is relatively safe, occasional accidents occur that lead to injury of the artery and make the circulation worse.

THE FOOT IN DANGER

Treatment for people with foot pain at rest is more difficult. Here it is imperative to do whatever is possible to improve the circulation because the leg is in great danger. Vasodilator drugs may help a little but generally not enough. In this situation, a bypass operation, if it is feasible, is best.

If you are unfortunate enough to have a leg amputated, you will understandably be depressed for a while. But there is much that can be done for you. Rehabilitation techniques have improved greatly in recent years, and your chances of walking again may be excellent. If your general strength is fairly good, you can be trained over a few weeks to use an artificial leg. Once you begin to walk with it, your gait will improve quickly and eventually be almost indistinguishable from anyone else's. In fact, many people with two amputations are walking about normally without anyone being aware of their condition.

AORTIC ANEURYSMS

Arteries tend to lose their elasticity as we grow older. They get stiffer and so do not tolerate as well the pressure of the blood as it flows through.

The walls of these stiffening arteries may gradually be pushed outward with each heartbeat, and they cannot snap back. This widening, if it occurs throughout an artery, poses no real danger. But a widening in a limited area (*aneurysm*) is dangerous. If one section of the arterial tree becomes wider than the rest, a delicate balance is upset, and the artery may rupture with massive bleeding.

Aneurysms develop most often where an artery branches sharply, causing the blood to press heavily against the wall as it goes around the curve. The sharpest branching point in the human body is the end of the major artery (aorta) at the point where it branches into the arteries to each leg. As a result, the terminal aorta in the abdomen is the most common site for an aneurysm (fig. 4).

This aortic aneurysm is insidious and extremely dangerous. It has been estimated that one out of every two hundred and fifty people over the age of fifty die of aortic aneurysm rupture. Unfortunately, this rupture tends to occur suddenly and without warning in much the same way as a tire blowing out at high speed on a highway. Your doctor can find evidence of the aneurysm before it blows. When he examines your abdomen, he can feel a strong pulsation.

If diagnosed before it ruptures, the aneurysm can be easily repaired with surgery. Periodic physical checkups could save thousands of lives every year by picking up aneurysms more frequently in their early stages.

We now have a new test called *ultrasound*, which can diagnose aneurysms correctly in almost every case. In this test, high frequency sound waves are aimed at the abdomen in the direction of the aorta, and the reflected waves coming back to a recording machine give an accurate picture of the location, size, and shape of the aorta. The test is simple, painless, and safe, and shows promise of becoming a good tool for screening large numbers of asymptomatic people for the presence or absence of aortic aneurysm. Your doctor will most likely order this test if he has any doubts about whether you do or do not have an aneurysm.

BLOOD CLOTS AND ANEURYSMS

In an aneurysm, the blood flow slows down. This leads to clotting. The clotting problem occurs frequently in the second most common aneurysm, which develops behind the knee (*popliteal aneurysm*). This aneurysm occurs because

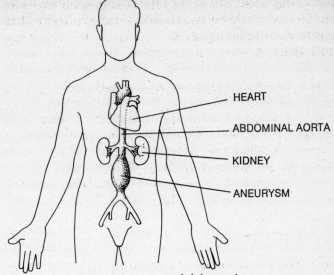

HEART

ABDOMINAL AORTA

KIDNEY

ANEURYSM

Fig. 4   Aneurysm of abdominal aorta.

the popliteal artery is subject to chronic stretching injury when we flex and extend our knees. It is particularly common in people such as house painters and mechanics who must bend a lot in their work.

The popliteal aneurysm is usually silent until a major clot occurs that may lead to loss of the leg. The clot travels down the leg and clogs the arteries. Just as in the case of aortic aneurysms, your doctor can find a popliteal aneurysm on careful, routine examination. This aneurysm can be simply and safely repaired by a surgical procedure. This should be done as soon as the aneurysm is discovered and before clots form.

SLOWING DOWN ARTERIOSCLEROSIS

At present arteriosclerosis cannot be prevented. But we know about some of the things that bring it on—and we can do something about these. We're not sure how much these factors contribute, or why certain individuals get arteriosclerosis earlier than others, or why it comes on faster in some and slower in others. But experts agree that you will be protected from arteriosclerosis for a longer time if you can avoid the following.

HIGH BLOOD PRESSURE (HYPERTENSION)

Sustained high blood pressure makes arteries age more rapidly. Blockage of arteries to the legs, heart, and brain occurs earlier in people who have hypertension. This holds even more strikingly for aneurysms. Fortunately, almost all hypertension can be well controlled with medication (see Chapter 6 for a full discussion of hypertension).

FATS IN THE BLOOD

Overweight and the elevation of certain fatty substances in the blood, such as cholesterol and triglycerides, seem to hasten the hardening of your arteries. Both of these factors are more common in affluent societies and result from overeating in general and from diets high in saturated fats. Many authorities believe that you can reduce the risk of arteriosclerosis by limiting the amount of whole-milk products, red meat, candies, and cakes in your diets and, equally important, by keeping track of the total number of calories you consume every day. An excellent goal to shoot for is to keep your adult weight within five pounds of your weight at full maturity (about age twenty-five).

SMOKING

If you're a smoker, stop. If you're not, don't start. We don't know everything about the effects of smoking on the body. But we know enough, and what we know tells us that:

1. Smoking harms your arteries. The nicotine in cigarettes causes spasms of the arteries.
2. Burning tobacco gives off carbon monoxide, which interferes with oxyen getting to the cells of your body.

3. Smokers have more lung cancer, heart attacks, strokes, and limb amputations than nonsmokers.

We can't think of a single good reason for smoking. Any way you look at it, smoking is harmful, more harmful to some than to others, but harmful to everybody. It kills many people.

If you value your arteries, don't smoke.

DIABETES

People with diabetes (high blood sugar, see Chapter 7) are likely to develop arteriosclerosis at an earlier age than people who do not have diabetes. We do not know exactly why this is so. Unfortunately, medication to lower the blood-sugar level does not prevent arteriosclerosis. Of the risk factors that we have mentioned, diabetes is the only one that is probably not preventable.

SUMMARY

1. Poor circulation in the legs is a common problem for older people, but most do not have symptoms. So have regular physical checkups and be sure your doctor looks for signs of arteriosclerosis in your legs. It's easy to detect. Good foot care can prevent serious problems from developing.

2. An aortic aneurysm is a silent time bomb in many older people. Careful, regular checkups can pick this up, and surgery can repair it.

3. There are a few things that you can do to slow down hardening of the arteries:

a) Have your blood pressure checked regularly, at least yearly.
b) Do not smoke.
c) Stay trim. Keep your weight down.
d) Avoid saturated fats in your diet.

2

HEART ATTACKS: FACTS CAN MEET YOUR FEARS

Most people are alarmed when they experience any unusual feelings in their chests. They assume that something has gone wrong with their hearts. Sometimes, of course, they are quite right. But not all chest pains mean heart trouble. The chest, like every other part of the body, is composed of many different parts: muscle, bone, nerves, the lungs, and the heart. Any one of these organs may cause chest pains. Indeed, there are just as many reasons for pain in the chest as there are for leg cramps, stomachache, or headache.

In this chapter we shall be dealing with one of the very common causes of chest pains: heart disease. But first let us see how the heart functions and why, under certain conditions, it produces characteristic symptoms.

THE HEART'S BLOOD SUPPLY

Just like an engine, the human body cannot function unless it is supplied with energy. This energy comes to us in the blood the heart pumps to every cell in the body. The heart pumps blood to itself, too, through the coronary arteries.

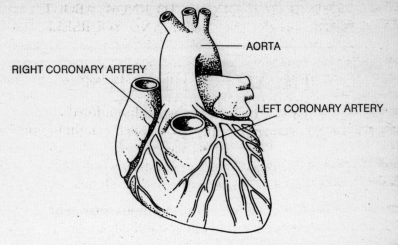

Fig. 5   Coronary arteries. These supply blood to the heart muscle.

When hardening of the arteries (arteriosclerosis, see page 4) develops, the coronary arteries become clogged, and the flow of blood to one or more areas of the heart's muscle decreases. The individual may then develop symptoms caused by poor oxygen supply (*ischemia*), and he is then said to have coronary heart disease.

ANGINA

The most common symptom of coronary heart disease is pain in the chest, which usually has characteristic qualities and is called *angina pectoris*. Since the heart needs more oxygen when it has to work harder, angina pectoris generally occurs during exertion of some kind, such as lifting a heavy package, walking rapidly, running, or climbing stairs. The pain is promptly relieved (within five to ten minutes) by rest. The more serious the heart disease is, the sooner the feeling of pain with any exertion comes on. For this reason, a doctor will ask the person with heart disease how many blocks he can walk or how many steps he can climb before he experiences pain.

In some cases, the exertion that brings on angina may not be very obvious. Anxiety, anger, frustration, or other forms of emotional tension tax the heart and can cause chest pains. Some people have chest pain mostly when they are in bed (*angina decubitus*). Anginal pain may also be due to the agitation aroused during a dream. In general, however, when angina, which has previously occurred only with physical activity, begins to occur when a person is resting or exerting himself only slightly, his heart condition is probably worsening.

THE PAIN OF ANGINA PECTORIS

Angina pectoris may appear in a number of different ways, most often as a tightness or compression or like a weight on the middle of the chest. Some individuals feel it as a stabbing or knifelike chest pain that leaves them breathless. Many people with angina experience difficulty in breathing rather than actual pain. On the other hand, a numbness or burning pain in the chest is rarely related to heart disease.

It is most important to keep in mind that the pain of angina is entirely *inside* the chest. It does not affect the outside structures of the chest like ribs, muscles, and skin. There is no external tenderness associated with anginal pain. Thus, if pressing or touching your chest causes pain, it is exceedingly unlikely that you are suffering from the pain of heart disease.

The third characteristic of angina pectoris is its location. It usually occurs in the mid-chest and feels as though it is coming from just behind the breastbone (sternum). (A doctor would refer to it as substernal or restrosternal pain.) A small number of people experience their angina in an unusual location, such as the neck, mid-back, left rib cage area, and even upper abdomen. A tightening pain in the neck that comes on with exertion and subsides with rest may be angina rather than arthritis. Pain in the upper abdomen that occurs during emotional stress in a tense individual may occasionally be angina rather than a stomach ulcer. Angina in any given person always occurs in the same place and occurs rather consistently with a given amount of exertion or stress. If chest pains occur in different parts of the chest area or are brought on by different stimuli, the chances are they are not being caused by heart disease.

HOW ANGINAL PAIN TRAVELS

The fourth characteristic of angina is the radiation, or traveling, of the pain. Typically, anginal pain moves from the mid-chest across the upper left side of the chest into the left shoulder and down the left arm. In fact, the pain is called angina pectoris because it passes through the upper chest (pectoral) muscles on the way to the left shoulder.

We really do not know much about the factors that determine how and where pain travels, but we do know that it has something to do with the pathway of nerves as they enter and leave the spinal cord. The heart sits in the chest

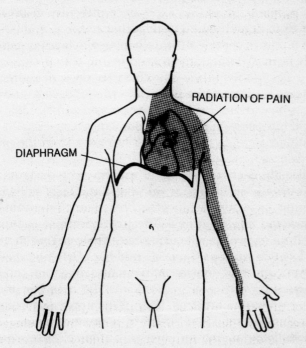

Fig. 6   Radiation of pain with heart attacks or angina.

just on top of the left diaphragm, and the nerve that controls the movement of the diaphragm branches out from the spinal cord in close proximity to the entrance of the nerves carrying sensation from the left shoulder and arm. In some mysterious way, the circuits seem to become crossed so that heart pain, through the nerve supply of the diaphragm, can cause pain in the left shoulder.

Disease or inflammation in other structures near the left diaphragm can also cause pain radiating to the left shoulder, and may be confused with angina pectoris. For example, a distended stomach or protrusion of the stomach into the chest through a weakness in the diaphragm (hiatus hernia) may mimic angina very closely. Infection in the abdomen under the diaphragm or surrounding the left lung just above the diaphragm can do the same thing.

Just as the nature and location of angina can be atypical, so can the radiation. Some people experience angina that radiates to the right shoulder, the back, or the neck. Others have radiation to the lower arm and wrist, skipping the shoulder. In fact, some people describe pain in the left wrist radiating to the chest. In many cases, there is no pain radiation at all. All of these patterns may be due to many other diseases or minor ailments, but the possibility of angina must always be considered.

NITROGLYCERINE: A MAGIC MEDICINE

The final characteristic of angina is its remarkable response to a drug called *nitroglycerine*. This drug in tablet form is placed under the tongue and rapidly absorbed by the body without being swallowed. Within a few minutes (usually two to three minutes), angina pectoris disappears in most cases. For many years, no one really understood why this drug worked so remarkably well. In recent years, however, special X-ray procedures have shown that nitroglycerine actually dilates (opens up) some of the healthy coronary arteries and their branches so that they can bring blood to the areas of the heart normally supplied by the clogged arteries. In addition, the nitroglycerine dilates other arteries in the body so that the heart has less work to do in pumping blood through them. No other pain responds to nitroglycerine in this dramatic way.

WHAT TO DO ABOUT CHEST PAINS

In short, your doctor has five important characteristics to consider in making a diagnosis of angina pectoris: relation to exertion, quality of pain, location, radiation, and response to nitroglycerine. Although we have already pointed out that any of these characteristics may be atypical or absent in some cases, at least three or four are necessary to make the diagnosis. Doctors consider its relation to exertion and its response to nitroglycerine the most important features of angina.

If you have any kind of pain or discomfort somewhere between the neck and upper abdomen, if the discomfort occurs regularly and consistently with exertion or emotional stress and is relieved promptly by rest, see your doctor at once.

Your doctor will take a careful history, examine you, and then most probably take an electrocardiogram. The electrocardiogram is a record of the electrical impulses going through the heart and gives a great deal of information about the condition of the heart muscle.

If an electrocardiogram is taken during an attack of angina pectoris, it will almost always show abnormalities. However, many people with coronary heart disease have normal electrocardiograms between attacks of angina.

In this situation, doctors often employ an exercise test during which you may be walking on a treadmill, pumping on a stationary bicycle, or walking up and down a short flight of steps. While you are exercising, the doctor is carefully watching your electrocardiogram. If certain changes occur, your doctor can be quite sure that you have some kind of coronary heart disease.

ACTIVITY LIMITS

A person with angina needs encouragement and guidance. He gradually learns by experience how much activity he can tolerate without pain, but he needs help in determining how far or how much he should exert himself. This decision also depends on his age, general health, and life-style. We have learned that people with angina can do a great deal. In fact, some doctors encourage their patients to take nitroglycerine before certain activities, such as sexual intercourse, in order to prevent pain. In many cases, the doctor and patient, working together, can develop an exercise program to strengthen the heart and perhaps decrease or even eliminate angina.

WHAT IS A HEART ATTACK?

If angina is pain caused by lack of blood supply to the heart, what is a heart attack? A heart attack (myocardial infarction) occurs when the clogging of an artery becomes worse in one area of the heart. If an area of the heart receives so little oxygen that it cannot manage to maintain itself at all, it may suddenly die. Its cells can no longer function or maintain their strength. That part of the heart muscle ceases to pump and degenerates into a soft, flabby material that is later replaced by scar tissue (fig. 7).

The heart attack may occur because an artery that is partially blocked becomes completely clogged by a blood clot that forms on its diseased walls, or a small portion of heart muscle may suddenly die without any change in the artery that feeds it. In this case, the attack occurs because the heart has been taxed beyond the capacity of a partially clogged artery to supply blood. This latter mechanism explains why people have heart attacks so often during or shortly after extreme emotional stress or exertion that is unusual for them. A familiar example of this kind of heart attack occurs in the relatively sedentary middle-aged man, who goes out to shovel his walk on a cold winter day and develops severe chest pain or even suddenly dies. Some doctors believe that a heart attack can occur even when the coronary arteries are normal if the physical strain is great enough. This is one explanation given for the occasional

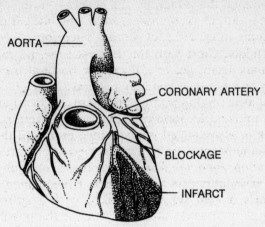

AORTA

CORONARY ARTERY

BLOCKAGE

INFARCT

Fig. 7   Heart after a heart attack. Note that the blockage in the coronary artery has led to damage to the area of heart muscle which it feeds.

athlete who develops a heart attack in the midst of severe, competitive activities, such as basketball and track.

DIAGNOSIS OF HEART ATTACKS

The typical heart attack causes a severe, crushing kind of pain behind the breastbone. This pain may or may not radiate to the left shoulder and arm. Like angina, it may be described as a pressing and severe heaviness on the chest, but it is generally much more severe than angina and does not respond promptly to either rest or nitroglycerine. The pain often lasts for several hours unless relieved by an injection of a painkiller such as demerol or morphine. However, this does not always happen this way. A heart attack may cause severe or mild pain and occasionally even occur without pain.

The electrocardiograms of many older people show evidence of scars that occurred after heart attacks even though these people cannot remember having had any pain. These incidents are often called "silent" heart attacks. Other people may have a mild twinge in the middle of the chest that they ascribe to indigestion. Unfortunately, one cannot judge the seriousness of the attack by the severity of the symptoms. Every heart attack is potentially fatal, and one cannot predict the outcome in the first few hours. Therefore, if you experience a sudden chest pain for the first time, no matter how mild it may seem, get to a doctor or hospital immediately. You may be having, or you may just have had, a heart attack.

Just as in angina pectoris, the pain of a heart attack may have an unusual location or radiation. A severe pain in the mid-back or a prolonged, unexplained cramp in the neck or arm in some people can be the first sign of a heart attack. In this situation, there are sometimes other symptoms that suggest the possibility of a heart attack. Unexplained sweating, particularly a cold sweat associated with a suffocating or pressing pain, should make you think of the possibility of a heart attack even if the pain is not in the chest. Again, get immediate medical attention.

Sometimes, a heart attack causes a steady pain in the upper abdomen, nausea, and even vomiting. What seems like acute indigestion can be much more serious. On the other hand, if you also have diarrhea and/or abdominal cramps, your problem is not likely to be related to the heart. Call for medical help if you have any unusual indigestion.

THE HEART ATTACK FOLLOWING ANGINA

Thus far in our discussion of heart attacks, we have been describing the individual who has a sudden, unexpected heart attack without any prior history of coronary heart disease. This is the most common way in which heart attacks present themselves. But a large number of people who get heart attacks have had angina pectoris. These people often have difficulty in deciding whether they are having just another anginal attack or an actual heart attack. Not infrequently, even a doctor may require three or four days of electrocardiograms and blood tests in order to distinguish between the two. There are several reasons for this difficulty. First, in a given individual, the pain of angina may be quite similar to the heart attack pain. In fact, many people with angina may not even suspect that they have had a heart

attack until an electrocardiogram taken at their next sched-
uled visit to the doctor shows signs of damage to their heart.

Although heart attack pain does not usually disappear
quickly with rest or administration of nitroglycerine, people
with previous angina may sometimes obtain some relief from
nitroglycerine even when they are having a heart attack or
just about to have one.

In some cases, an increase in the frequency of angina
and a decrease in the exertion required to bring it on may be
a warning of an impending heart attack. Inside the chest, a
coronary artery may be gradually closing down completely,
and within a few days, the patient may actually experience
the more severe and prolonged pain of a typical heart attack.

Another warning sign to a person with angina is the
diminishing effectiveness of his nitroglycerine. If he does not
obtain prompt relief from pain with his usual dose of nitroglycerine (usually one tablet) or a maximum of one additional tablet, he should see a doctor immediately.

A similar cause for concern is an increase in the time it
takes to get relief from rest or nitroglycerine. ·A person
whose attacks begin to last twenty minutes instead of five
minutes may be about to have a heart attack. (*Caution*: If
the response to nitroglycerine is inadequate, the worst thing
to do is to continue to take one tablet after another. This
overdosage will result in so much opening of the arteries in
the lower portion of the body that too much blood will flow
to these areas and the person will faint.) Here again—see a
doctor immediately.

USE AND ABUSE OF NITROGLYCERINE

Nitroglycerine tablets have a very short shelf life. They are
what the chemists call an unstable compound, and they lose
their effectiveness after about two to three months. Frequently, old, outdated tablets do not relieve angina. In fact,
doctors whose patients complain of chest pains not relieved
by medication sometimes forget to ask them how long they
have had their nitroglycerine tablets, and so they are misled
in their diagnoses of the cause of the chest pains.

RISK FACTORS FOR CORONARY HEART DISEASE

Although no one knows just how arteriosclerosis begins and gradually clogs the coronary and other arteries throughout the body, we have learned a lot in recent years about some of the factors that cause clogging in the coronary arteries. Some of these factors are inherited and therefore beyond our control, but there are definitely a number of things that we can do to slow down hardening of the arteries and perhaps prevent angina and heart attacks.

SMOKING

All of the available evidence tells us that smoking plays a significant part in the development of coronary heart disease. Once a person has this disease, there is convincing evidence that smoking of cigarettes makes angina worse and increases the possibility of sudden death. Since we do not know precisely what substances in tobacco damage the arterial walls, there is little reason to think that filtering the cigarettes will make a significant difference. We must first know what has to be filtered out. In addition to the damage done by unknown substances in tobacco, we know nicotine tends to constrict arteries. A sudden narrowing of an already damaged artery can lead to a heart attack and even sudden death. There may be a role, therefore, for lower-nicotine cigarettes for totally addicted people who cannot seem to stop smoking. There is no question, however, about the best and only thing people with coronary disease must do: *stop smoking entirely*. Smoking is harmful to everyone. For the person with heart disease, smoking has serious and sometimes fatal consequences.

DIET AND WEIGHT

Diet is an important factor in coronary heart disease. Too many of us eat too much and too many rich foods. The results are clear and inevitable. Obesity, particularly obesity acquired in the adult years, is closely linked to coronary heart disease. Several studies have shown that the closer your weight remains to what it was at age twenty-five, the less chance you have of getting a heart attack. People who go through adult life without becoming more than five pounds heavier have only a very small chance of ever having a heart attack. Of course, it is not easy in a sedentary society to keep your weight down to a gain of about one-sixth of a pound per year over a thirty- or forty-year-period, but it can be done.

Most overweight people consume large amounts of saturated fats found in such foods as fatty meats, butter, whole milk, and cream products, and deep-fried foods. These people have a high incidence of coronary heart disease. This is true throughout the world. In Japan, for example, the diet is low in saturated fats. The Japanese have fewer heart attacks than we Americans. However, when Japanese emigrate to the United States and change their eating habits, they get more heart attacks than the Japanese at home. We find that as a nation becomes more industrialized and more affluent, its people increasingly add *solid fat* in the form of meat and luxury foods to their diets. And, at the same time, they get more heart attacks.

DIETARY ADVICE

We suggest you follow these prudent dietary suggestions:

1. Eat more poultry and less beef.
2. Eat your beef well done rather than rare. Well-done beef has had some of its fats burned off in the cooking process.
3. Drink skimmed milk or low-fat milk.
4. Avoid butter and eat cheese sparingly. Skimmed-milk cheeses are preferable.
5. Eliminate egg yolks entirely, or limit yourself to one or two eggs a week.
6. Avoid deep-fat frying.
7. Fry only with unsaturated cooking oils such as corn oil and peanut oil. Avoid deep frying because this converts unsaturated fat to saturated fat.
8. Cut out or minimize eating of sweets.

HYPERTENSION

A third important factor in the development of coronary heart disease is hypertension (high blood pressure, see Chapter 6). It has been estimated that at least 10 percent (about 20 million people) of the United States population has hypertension, although very few have symptoms of coronary heart disease. Hypertensive people suffer more heart attacks and strokes than the rest of the population. On the positive side, however, doctors now have at their disposal a variety of relatively safe drugs with which to treat this disease. Practically all hypertension is controllable if a patient and his doctor work together. However, to treat hypertension, one must first detect it. You should have your blood pressure checked periodically.

EXERCISE

Many studies have provided rather strong statistical proof that regular physical activity is of value in preventing heart attacks. One of the earliest and most interesting studies involved the London bus drivers and conductors. The drivers sat at the wheel throughout the workday, while the conductors moved around constantly as they checked the tickets of passengers. Health records of a large group of drivers and conductors were studied and matched according to age, smoking habits, and other risk factors. The investigators found that the more sedentary bus drivers had more heart attacks than conductors of the same age in whom the other risk factors were similar. Just the constant walking of the conductors seemed to make a difference. This kind of study has been repeated in other groups, including American longshoremen, with the same results.

A recently published study of the life-style of Harvard graduates confirmed the value of strenuous exercise. Those graduates who performed vigorous exercise on a regular basis for many years had, on the average, fewer heart attacks and a longer life span that the less active group. In this study, light exercise such as walking and golf did not seem to help. More vigorous activities such as jogging, basketball, and tennis seemed to be the key.

It seems clear that we would all benefit from a prudent, regular program of physical activity, especially if our jobs keep us pretty much chained to our desks. If your job is a sedentary one, you might benefit from some kind of provision for exercise in your leisure hours. This can take the form of competitive games or workouts in a gymnasium, but jogging will do just as well to keep you in trim.

Here, caution is in order. Don't become a weekend athlete. You may do yourself more harm than good if you suddenly put a heavy strain on your heart. If you are middle-aged or older and you haven't been doing much physical exercise, you must gradually condition your body and your circulation to meet the additional strain of strenuous exercise. Any physical activity which makes heavy demands on you (tennis, swimming, and jogging) must be started slowly and gradually, especially if you are over fifty-five and have not been physically active for a long period of time. Before you take up any program of strenuous physical activity, see your doctor. Ask him to check you thoroughly to determine whether it is safe for you. Even if you have no symptoms, an exercise test may be advisable to make sure that your heart is normal and able to stand the strain of vigorous exercise.

Less strenuous activities, such as walking and golf, usually present no problem. You can start them on your own, but it may be a good idea to see a doctor first anyway. Although the specific value of light exercise in preventing heart attacks is still a point of dispute, these activities will certainly help keep you trim, leaner, and more relaxed. This, in itself, has some protective value.

But no matter what kind of program you decide to follow, keep this in mind. The key word in a safe and successful program is *moderation*.

PSYCHOLOGICAL PROFILE

We don't know for sure, but there is some reason to believe that the hard-driving, high-strung, goal-oriented, very competitive individual who doesn't know how to relax and enjoy his leisure time may be more prone to heart attacks than the more relaxed, less tense individual. This is one explanation advanced for the frequency of heart attacks in high-ranking business executives.

If you are constantly worrying, driving yourself, not getting enough rest and relaxation, take a good, hard look at yourself. Without interfering with your daily activities, you can begin to change your attitudes toward yourself and your job. You can begin to reduce some of your internal and external pressures. You may not be able to do this with all your pressures, but you can generally do something to make your life less stressful and thus reduce the chances of your getting a heart attack.

DIABETES MELLITUS

For many reasons (see chapter 7), diabetics as a group tend to have more heart attacks than nondiabetics. At present, the individual has little or no control over whether he will or won't get diabetes. We have learned much about some of the causes of diabetes, but still do not fully understand why or how it attacks some people and not others.

ADJUSTMENT TO HEART DISEASE

You've had a heart attack and you have recovered. What will the rest of your life be like? Of course, much will depend on how severely the attack has damaged your heart, and how quickly you adjust to some of the new realities you must face. But, under proper medical care, you should be able to do most and perhaps all of the things you did before. You can expect that you may have to limit your activities somewhat in some areas.

In most instances, only a very small area of your heart will not be functioning, but the rest of your heart will make up for this loss.

Here are some things you can do while you are getting your strength back.

1. In the very beginning, you may feel quite depressed and discouraged. You may be wondering whether you'll ever be able to live a normal, useful life again. It's natural for you to feel this way, but don't allow yourself to remain in this mood. It could very well be more disabling than the heart attack itself. Don't bury your feelings. Talk to your doctor, your friends, your family. Look around at others who have had heart attacks and are now functioning well, and listen to them rather than to your own fears.

2. From time to time, you may experience anginal pains. Your doctor will tell you what they mean and how you should deal with them. Above all, don't focus your attention on your chest. If you do, you are sure to become aware of all kinds of subtle sensations you may have never been aware of before. Some people literally disable themselves this way. Their fear of getting another heart attack becomes a sort of obsession, and so they avoid any exertion, even the most minimal. We know it is easier said than done, but you must turn your attention outward to the world, to your work, to your friends and family, to the normal activities you were involved in before your heart attack. Your doctor will tell you how to distinguish real from imaginary or unrelated symptoms and he'll tell you how to deal with them.

3. It generally takes a few months for people to increase their activities up to their full potential. Then you will want the answers to some very real, important questions. No two people are the same. No two heart attacks are the same. No two people have the same problems adjusting to their new and somewhat altered lives. So don't be afraid to ask your doctor.

Here is a list of some of the more common questions you will want answers to:

1. When can I walk outside of my house?
2. When can I climb stairs?
3. How far can I walk?

4. When can I have sexual intercourse?
5. Can I participate in athletics such as jogging, tennis, and golf?
6. Can I return to my previous occupation?
7. When can I return to work?
8. What kind of diet do I need?
9. Will I have more chest pains?
10. What should I do if I develop chest pains?

COMPLICATIONS OF CORONARY HEART DISEASE

SEVERE PAIN

Some people with coronary disease develop more complex problems that may require close medical attention and medication. The most common complication relates to angina. Chest pain may become disabling, occurring at rest or with minimal activity. Some people with severe angina cannot walk more than a few steps or lift a bag of groceries. Control of hypertension, reduction in weight, and cessation of smoking may decrease these symptoms considerably. If the angina is still severe, a medication called propranolol may provide further relief by making the heart work less. Since both the frequency and force of the heartbeat diminish, patients with severely damaged heart muscle cannot take this medication because it might cause fluid to back up in the lungs (see chapter 3). Once you start taking propranolol, it is dangerous to discontinue it without first checking with your doctor.

If your angina remains unrelieved despite these measures, your doctor may want to look into the possibility of surgery for the coronary arteries. In many cases, it is possible to perform a bypass graft. In this operation, the surgeon attaches a vein graft from your leg to the main artery of the body (aorta) and to the coronary artery beyond the clogged segment in the same way that a plumber replaces a corroded pipe. Most patients may require two or more such grafts.

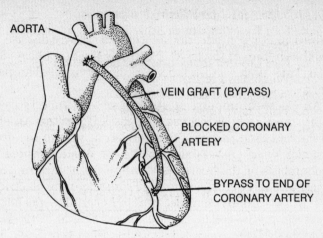

Fig. 8 Coronary bypass graft. The inserted graft brings blood to the coronary artery beyond the blockage.

Because of improved techniques in surgery and anesthesiology, it is possible to perform this operation in carefully selected cases with very few complications.

In order to determine whether a patient should have surgery, a cardiologist must perform a test called *coronary arteriography*. A special dye must be injected into these arteries through a tube placed in the main artery of the body (aorta). X-rays are then taken to determine how extensive the arterial blockage is. If the areas of clogging are relatively short, the bypass operation can be performed.

A DAMAGED PUMP

A heart attack may sometimes cause so much damage to the muscle that it cannot pump properly any longer. If the heart muscle fails in its pumping action, the major organs of the body do not receive enough blood and oxygen, and blood may back up into the lungs and other areas. The patient becomes short of breath, develops swollen legs, and may become confused. The doctor will usually prescribe Digitalis to strengthen the heart's pumping action and a diuretic pill to help the kidneys eliminate excess fluid (see chapter 3).

ERRATIC HEART RHYTHM

The third major complication of coronary heart disease involves the rhythm of the heart. Normally the heart beats at a regular rate under stimulation of its own reliable pacemakers.

An electrical impulse starts in a small structure called the *sinus node*, which is located in the left atrium. An electrical current then passes across the left atrium to the *atrioventricular node* (A-V Node), which is situated where all four chambers of the heart (left atrium, right atrium, right ventricle and left ventricle) meet. From there the electricity passes in an orderly manner through certain specialized conducting paths called *Bundle Branches* and *Purkinje fibers* to the heart muscle of the left and right ventricles. The heart muscle, on being stimulated, moves synchronously to create the pumping motion of each heartbeat.

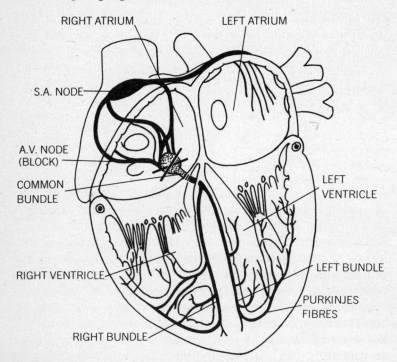

Fig. 9   Conducting system of the heart.

With advancing age and the development of arteri-osclerosis, these pacemakers may fail to function properly, resulting in irregular and erratic heart rhythm. These erratic rhythms are called *arrhythmias* and may be present all the time or only once in a while. They may cause the heart to beat too slowly or too quickly, or to have occasional extra beats (premature ventricular beats).

Many people having intermittent arrhythmias are free of symptoms, particularly those with premature ventricular beats. Others may have spells of palpitation, dizziness, feeling of weakness, or fainting episodes. If you have one of these complaints, see your doctor at once. He will check your electrocardiogram. If the electrocardiogram is normal, he may ask you to wear a special small monitoring device on your chest for twenty-four or forty-eight hours. As you go through your normal daily schedule, this device will contin-uously record your heartbeat. The doctor can review this and see whether you have any arrhythmias. If you have frequent premature ventricular beats, your doctor will pre-scribe an anti-arrhythmic drug like: quinidine, procainea-mide, or Norpace (disopyramide).

Treatment for these beats is important even if you have no symptoms because they can lead to a very dangerous arrhythmia called *ventricular tachycardia*. These beats are very common after heart attacks, and many doctors feel that every heart attack patient should have a twenty-four-hour monitoring before going home, and perhaps a few months after the heart attack.

Although the anti-arrhythmic drugs are effective and generally quite safe, side effects sometimes occur. Quinidine occasionally destroys many of the blood's platelets. These cells enable the blood to clot. Without them, bleeding may occur anywhere in the body, most commonly in the skin. If "black-and-blue" marks or little blue dots appear on the skin, see your doctor right away. Procainamide may lead to joint pains, rashes, chest pains, and fever. Norpace may make it difficult for men with large prostate glands to pass urine. All of these symptoms go away quickly when the guilty drug is stopped.

Pacemakers

If your heart tends to beat too slowly, you may need an artificial pacemaker. The invention of the artificial pacemaker has saved thousands of lives during the last twenty years. This device has been gradually improved during that space of time and is now very safe and reliable. The pacemaker functions only when your own pacemaker doesn't work. It is set to keep the heart beating at a certain rate so that it turns on when the heart goes below that rate and turns off when the heart goes above that rate.

Insertion of the pacemaker into the body is very simple. The entire procedure can be performed with local anesthesia and is one of the safest procedures in all of surgery. A wire is passed through a vein in the arm into the heart (right ventricle). The power pack supplying electric current is placed under the skin of the chest and hooked up to the wire. The chest itself is not opened.

When pacemakers were first invented, the power packs had to be replaced within two years, but the newer models generally last for a much longer time. In fact, new lithium power packs can be expected to last as long as ten years. When the power pack begins to wear out, it is very easily replaced with a small cut in the skin under local anesthesia.

Since some power packs wear out sooner than others, you must be seen regularly by your cardiologist. He will check your electrocardiogram and also use a minicomputer to make sure that the pacemaker is precisely on schedule.

During the first two or three years, you will probably need to see him every six months and as the power pack ages, you may have to go more often, perhaps every three months. If you should have any spells of weakness or dizziness or a fainting episode, you should not wait for the next visit. Check with your doctor immediately, and if he is not available, go to the nearest hospital emergency room.

Many people are concerned about the quality of their lives after pacemaker insertion. This concern is totally unnecessary because you can lead a perfectly normal life with an artificial pacemaker. It does not preclude any of your normal activities. There may be some restrictions on your activities because of your heart disease and angina, but the pacemaker does not add to them. For example, people ask whether they can go swimming with a pacemaker. Of course, the answer is yes, as long as the cold water does not produce angina.

The only precautions you must take involve magnetic fields. A strong magnetic field can occasionally make the pacemaker speed up, forcing your heart to beat too quickly. Thus, it is a wise policy to avoid certain situations:

1. Do not go near microwave ovens and do not have one in your house. If you take an airplane trip, be sure that you are not seated near the kitchenette areas.
2. When you go to an airport, do not allow anyone to use a portable magnet to search you for metallic objects.
3. Stay away from industrial sources of magnetism, such as electromagnets and induction coils.

DRUGS TO PROTECT THE HEART

There is a growing body of evidence to suggest that certain drugs, which interfere with the blood's platelets, may have a protective effect against heart attacks. These platelets are involved in clotting of blood. Some authorities believe that simple aspirin as well as a drug called sulfinpyrazone may be good for some patients who have had heart attacks. You can discuss this possibility with your doctor.

SUMMARY

1. Coronary heart disease is one of the major afflictions of mankind.

2. Most chest pains are not related to the heart. Angina pectoris, which is due to clogged coronary arteries, usually occurs during exertion and is relieved promptly by rest and nitroglycerine.

3. A heart attack results from severe clogging of a coronary artery.

4. Most people can lead normal lives after a heart attack.

5. After a heart attack, do not be afraid to ask your physician detailed questions about what you can do and when you can do it.

6. If your angina pectoris becomes disabling, you may be a candidate for a coronary bypass operation. In selected cases, the results are excellent.

7. Certain risk factors for coronary heart disease can be avoided or treated:

    a) Avoid smoking
    b) Cut down on fatty foods
    c) Keep your weight down
    d) Have your blood pressure checked regularly
    e) Stay physically active.

3

SHORT-WINDEDNESS I:
THE HEART AS
THE CULPRIT

There is nothing unusual about panting for breath after a
frantic rush for the bus or a hurried sprint up a flight of
stairs. You expect it. But you don't expect it after a short
walk down the block.

It may seem inconceivable that this sensation which
you casually accept as normal after strenuous activity can
develop after such a simple exercise. But it does occur—and
is often a clue to an underlying ailment. Did you ever stop to
think just what shortness of breath really is? In simplest
terms, it is *actually feeling* yourself *breathing, knowingly
directing your own* breathing. Just try to recall any time
when your breathing was actually dependent on your conscious control of each breath. Obviously, breathing continues whether you think about it or not, but there are times
when it becomes necessary for us to appreciate or sense our
own breathing. This is nature's alert system that warns us of
a breakdown somewhere in the finely tuned system that
regulates our heart and lungs and the delivery of oxygen to
our body.

Before we discuss some of the problems that lead to
shortness of breath, we should understand how the heart
and lungs function.

OXYGEN, THE HEART, AND THE LUNGS

Your body is composed of countless cells, each of which leads an individual life, and each requires oxygen to survive. In a way, the life of these cells can be likened to the steady glow of a candle. The living flame consumes the wax, its food, and in so doing, gives off a waste product, the black carbon soot on the glass lamp. If we cover the flame and deprive it of oxygen, it goes out. In a similar way, the cells of your body require oxygen to consume or burn the food you provide, and in so doing, give off a waste product, carbon dioxide. But unlike the soot, this waste product is invisible. Since most of the cells of your body are not in direct contact with the oxygen in the air, this must be delivered to them. The red blood cells carry precious oxygen to these cells and remove the carbon dioxide. Propelled by the heart through miles of branching pipelines called *arteries* and *capillaries*, the blood reaches every cell of the body and returns through veins back to the heart.

In this complicated circuit, the lungs can be called the ventilation system of the blood. For before blood is delivered to the body, it must pass along a countless number of tiny air chambers called *alveoli*, where it acquires fresh oxygen and releases into these chambers the carbon dioxide it has received. The air that we inhale passes down our main windpipe through many branching smaller air tubes (*bronchi*) until it reaches these tiny air chambers that cluster about the air tubes like grapes on a single stem. Thus, blood acquires oxygen from these chambers, enters the heart, which sends it to all the cells of your body, and finally it returns again to the lungs.

The heart is a set of two separate pumps. One receives blood returning from the body and delivers it to the lungs. The other receives blood from the lungs and pumps it to the entire body.

Each pump is made up of a *ventricle* that does the pumping and an *atrium*, which is an antechamber for blood waiting to be pumped by the ventricle. The right pump

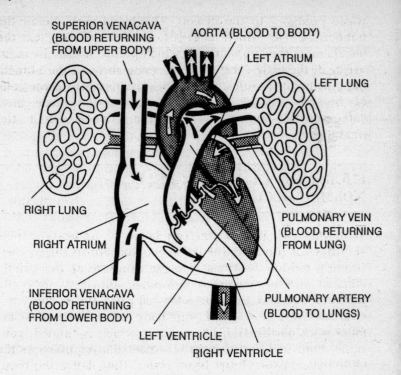

Fig. 10   Circulation of the blood through the heart.
1. Blood returning from the body enters the right atrium through large veins.
2. Blood then enters the right ventricle where it is pumped to the lungs via the pulmonary arteries.
3. Blood returns from the lungs (where it receives oxygen) through the pulmonary veins and enters the left atrium.
4. Blood flows from the left atrium to the left ventricle which pumps it into the aorta.
5. From the aorta, blood is distributed to the body through many arteries.

sends blood to the lungs, and the left one sends it to the main artery of the body called the aorta.

As shown in the diagram, we can follow the course of a drop of blood from any point in the cycle. Blood enters the right atrium and then goes to the right ventricle, which pumps it into the pulmonary artery, which takes it to the lungs. There it enters capillaries, through which it receives oxygen from the alveoli and gives off carbon dioxide (a waste product) to the alveoli. The blood then enters the pulmonary vein, which takes it to the left atrium. Next the blood enters the left ventricle, which pumps it into the main artery of the body (aorta). After going through the branching pipeline of arteries, it enters capillaries near some cells of the body. The blood gives the cells oxygen, takes their carbon dioxide and returns through a series of veins to the right atrium.

SHORTNESS OF BREATH AS A NORMAL OCCURRENCE

With this background you can begin to understand how shortness of breath develops. When you are resting or performing routine activities, you are unaware of the quietly efficient work of your heart and lungs since they are easily providing the oxygen your body requires. When you exercise, however, the cells of your body, particularly muscles, must work harder and, like a flame which is fanned, consume more fuel and oxygen. To meet the requirement for more oxygen, your heart beats faster, thus delivering more blood. Simultaneously, breathing becomes more rapid to increase the supply of oxygen and eliminate waste products such as carbon dioxide. Your mind now registers the sensation of actively participating in breathing.

Sometimes the need for oxygen seems more apparent to some people than to others. In part, this is related to regular exercise or conditioning. An athlete may walk several miles without experiencing difficulty in breathing while a sedentary worker may find a one-block walk taxing. In the case of the athlete, the gradual conditioning of the heart to deliver more blood and of the muscles to use oxygen more efficiently develops only after a period of training. It is normal for a person who does not do much exercise to develop shortness of breath after vigorous exertion. Thus, as your level of daily activity diminishes over the years, you can expect to breathe more heavily after attempting strenuous activity that seemed so easy in earlier years.

Severe emotional distress can also cause shortness of

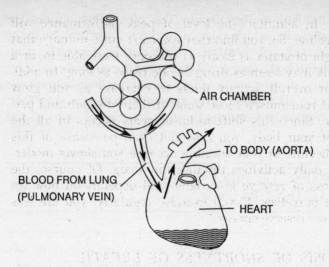

Fig. 11   Normal flow of blood from air chambers of lungs to heart (left side of heart).

breath. This is completely normal. The lover's sigh and the frightened gasp are nothing more than a form of momentary shortness of breath, in effect a gasp for oxygen. Emotional people, in particular, may breathe or sigh deeply and mistake this for a breathing problem. They are deliberately controlling their own breathing by thinking about their respiratory movements much as we do if we consciously attempt to control each breath. This condition is called *hyperventilation* and many of us may experience it in times of emotional crises or tragedy.

EFFECT OF AGE ON BREATHING

Normally, the heart and lungs have a reserve capacity that they can call upon in times of increased need, a sort of biological backup system. The heart delivers more blood at a swifter rate, and the lungs increase their efficiency according to our need for oxygen. As you grow older, you have less of this backup energy and are unable to respond to your needs as efficiently as before. Thus, even during normal activity, the heart and lungs may have to call upon their reserve strength. In addition, the level of peak performance will slowly decline. So, you find that you can't quite manage that extra flight of stairs as easily as you once were able to, or a short walk may seem as tiring as one twice as long. In addition, your overall activity tends to decrease as you grow older and your muscles lose some of their strength and performance. Since this shift to lower gears occurs in all the organs of your body, you may not even be aware of this gradual decline in your stamina because you slowly moderate your daily activities through the years. Of course, the rate of loss of reserve is variable and depends on how we condition ourselves. If you exercise regularly, you are less likely to lose reserve energy.

DIAGNOSIS OF SHORTNESS OF BREATH

If some shortness of breath is to be expected as you grow older, when should this be a cause of concern? In some instances the symptoms may develop so subtly and gradually that you are not aware that your pace has slowed. On the

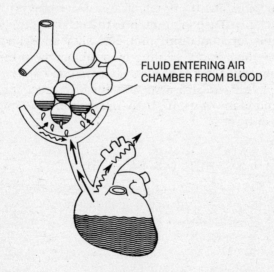

FLUID ENTERING AIR CHAMBER FROM BLOOD

Fig. 12   In congestive heart failure, the heart is unable to pump all the blood it receives from the lungs. Fluid from the backed-up blood seeps into the air chambers of the lungs.

other hand, abrupt onset of shortness of breath or short-windedness, which appears after less and less effort over a period of days or weeks, usually indicates a medical problem. This is also generally true for the occurrence of symptoms after minor activities that were previously considered routine. It may be as slight as having to stop at a landing of a staircase that, until recently, you could easily climb without rest. When other complaints accompany the shortness of breath, it is more likely that you have a physical problem. This is particularly so when cough, chest pain, blood in the sputum, or swelling of the legs appears. Once you recognize that you are having some difficulty breathing, see your doctor at once. There are many causes for shortness of breath.

SHORTNESS OF BREATH CAUSED BY HEART TROUBLE

A weakened heart may be unable to deliver an amount of blood that is adequate for the needs of the body. This condition is called *heart failure*. This is not as bad as it sounds. It indicates nothing more than that the heart fails to meet the demands that are made on it. That is, it does not quite pump a sufficient amount of blood for a particular level of activity. Because the amount of blood may not be adequate, less oxygen reaches the cells. The shortness of breath that appears is the message from the cells that they are not receiving enough oxygen.

We have previously noted that the blood receives its oxygen from the tiny air chambers of the lung and then streams through multiple rivulets to converge in the heart, which then pumps it to the entire body (fig. 11). When the heart weakens, it pumps less blood with each beat. Nevertheless, blood continues to pour into it from the lungs. With less blood leaving the heart than entering, some blood will begin to collect behind the heart much as water will collect behind a dam. This dammed-up blood slowly accumulates within the lungs and congests them, which is why the condition is called *congestive heart failure* (fig. 12). With the pressure of backed-up blood, the multiple tiny air chambers of the lungs may begin to soak up fluid from the blood, further interfering with breathing. It is the sound made by the presence of fluid in the air chambers (*rales*) that the doctor listens for when he examines the chest with a stethoscope for signs of heart failure.

OTHER INDICATIONS OF HEART PROBLEMS

In addition to shortness of breath, a weakened heart may eventually lead to the accumulation of salt and water in the body. This water accumulation is often first detected by swelling of the ankles, a condition referred to as *edema*. Of course there are many other causes for swelling of the ankles besides heart failure, but the combination with shortness of breath is often an early clue. At first, this fluid can be absorbed during periods when the heart is resting, as during sleep, which explains why it may not be present after awakening in the morning and develops as the heart works harder during the day. Thus, the earliest symptom of heart failure even before shortness of breath, may be the need to urinate several times during the night. The body is getting rid of the fluid accumulated during the day.

Another sign may be the inability to lie comfortably on one pillow without becoming short-winded. Some people have acquired the habit early in life of using two or more pillows at night. For them, using one pillow may seem uncomfortable but it does not lead to difficulty in breathing that appears with early heart failure.

One of the more dramatic and at times terrifying events that may appear with congestive heart failure is the sudden awakening in the middle of the night with a sense of suffocation. Some people must even stand before an open window to relieve the breathing difficulty. This is referred to by physicians as *paroxysmal nocturnal dyspnea*, or PND, which literally means "sudden attack of shortness of breath at night." This probably results from some of the fluid seeping into the lungs that has accumulated in the body during the day.

Any of these symptoms is reason enough to seek medical help promptly.

Since there are many degrees of weakening of the heart muscle, the heart failure may be extremely mild and may develop only on extreme exertion. Thus, the heart may pump an adequate amount of blood to do routine chores, but not be able to meet the demands imposed by severe exertion. The presence of heart failure or shortness of breath due to "heart trouble" should not be taken to mean that your heart has ceased to function but rather that it doesn't quite measure up to every demand you make upon it. There is certainly no reason for you to live a life of inactivity. Proper treatment often restores vigor to a weakened heart, and allows you to pursue a very productive and active life.

SEVERE HEART FAILURE

Some cases of heart failure may be very severe, often to the point where even routine effort leads to symptoms. The most extreme form of heart failure is a condition called *acute pulmonary edema*.

As we have noted, with the pressure of dammed-up blood in the lung, fluid from the blood can ooze into the tiny air chambers of the lung. If the amount of fluid is extensive, and many of the air chambers are "flooded," severe shortness of breath will result. The condition is quite analogous to drowning, and the patient can be said to be drowning in his own body fluid. It can develop with alarming suddenness, often within minutes, although it may develop over a longer period. Needless to say, this is an emergency situation requiring immediate medical attention. Any abrupt onset of shortness of breath, particularly in a person known to have congestive heart failure may indicate the presence of pulmonary edema. Nevertheless, prompt treatment will rapidly clear the lungs and make it possible for you to live as you did before.

In many instances there is a recognizable cause for this event, such as excessive salt intake, infection, or failure to take medicines properly. On occasion, this may be the only indication of a heart attack, even when there is no chest pain.

CAUSES OF HEART FAILURE

The most common cause of heart failure is damage to the muscles of the heart caused by hardening of the arteries to the heart. (See chapter 1.)

High blood pressure can also eventually lead to heart failure. In patients with high blood pressure the heart must work harder to squeeze blood through the vessels of the body against that higher pressure. To accomplish this, the muscles of the heart enlarge, but in so doing gradually injure themselves. At some point they are no longer able to pump the blood adequately, heart muscles weaken, and heart failure follows. There are many other causes of heart failure, such as injury to the valves of the heart and abnormal beats of the heart, but common to all these is the limitation imposed on the heart that prevents it from pumping at its best level.

TREATMENT OF HEART FAILURE

The management of heart failure involves a cooperative effort between the physician and patient. Despite the availability of a number of effective medicines, the patient must actively participate in a balanced program of activity, diet, and medication.

As we have already pointed out, heart failure is a weakening of the muscles of the heart. The degree of weakness varies from individual to individual so that no narrow definition of the amount of permissible activity can be applied to everyone. In fact, in many people the loss of strength in the heart muscle may be so minimal that shortness of breath develops only after severe exertion, whereas in others even simple tasks prove to be a burden to the heart. Older patients who have slowly altered their pace of activity over the years may scarcely detect the symptoms of heart failure except under unusually stressful circumstances.

Each individual must look closely at his daily activities and avoid the kinds of activity that place a great strain on the heart. For example, a patient with mild heart failure should not take on the duties of a longshoreman, but certainly could work as a cabdriver. Under most circumstances the presence of heart failure should not lead a person to avoid normal activity. On the contrary, honest and detached appraisal will often reveal many time-consuming but fruitless physical activities and lead one to more balanced and meaningful life. In many instances the presence of heart failure will have no perceptible effect on one's life-style. For example, patients often hesitate to travel. Generally, a patient with well-controlled heart failure can travel by plane or bus but should omit many hours of sitting still without stretching his legs for a while.

Perhaps the most difficult part of the treatment program for a patient to accept is the change in diet. People with heart failure tend to accumulate fluid in their bodies. This accumulated fluid produces many of the troublesome symptoms of heart failure. So the aim of treatment is to prevent this fluid buildup. Since a person cannot retain fluid without retaining salt or "sodium chloride," consumption of salt must be limited. Today, powerful medications are available to assist the body in eliminating salt, but these cannot be totally relied upon to prevent the retention of water in every instance. Patients are frequently bewildered by the precise definition of the amount of salt that they are permitted. Here are a few suggestions that apply to most people:

1. Stick close to the exact amount of salt your doctor tells you your diet should contain. This usually means no extra salt added to cooked foods. Don't experiment. Don't cheat.

2. Don't add salt from the salt shaker to your food.

3. Avoid all highly salted foods such as salami, pickles, and ham. You may be one of those people who can tolerate a certain amount of salt, but don't push your good fortune too far. Eat as if you couldn't tolerate salt at all. It's safer for you if you do.

4. Whenever possible, use fresh or frozen vegetables. Canned vegetables usually have a high salt content. Always

check the label. You'll be surprised—as most people are—at the amount of salt it contains.

5. When you eat out, don't be bashful. Ask the waiter or maître d'hôtel whether salt is used in cooking the dish you've ordered. Most restaurants use salt in their cooking. So you'll be much better off if you order your meal without salt. Restaurants are quite familiar with this kind of request from their patrons who have heart failure or high blood pressure, and they will prepare your meal as you want it.

MEDICATIONS FOR HEART FAILURE

The two most widely used preparations in the treatment of heart failure are "water pills" and Digitalis. Your doctor will generally recommend one or both of these medications along with a salt-restricted diet to treat the heart failure. The "water pill" that he prescribes actually prevents the kidney from retaining salt, thus causing the body to lose salt and water in the urine. Often, when doctors prescribe certain water pills, or *diuretics* as they are called, they prescribe potassium medication or instruct patients to drink a lot of orange juice or eat bananas or other foods rich in potassium salts. The reason for this is that the body tends to eliminate potassium together with sodium salts in the urine and this can significantly reduce the amount of potassium in the body. A patient with low-body potassium may develop severe weakness. More importantly, this can lead to serious abnormalities in heart rhythm in patients taking digitalis.

Digitalis is a very important part of the treatment of heart failure. There are many varieties and brand names of Digitalis, but these preparations all work by strengthening the contraction of the heart and thus assist it in pumping more blood with each beat. The dosage of digitalis must be carefully regulated. It is generally taken daily, and for life, since the beneficial effect that digitalis exerts on the heart is maintained only so long as the individual takes this medication.

Digitalis can be harmful if too much of it accumulates in the body. So it is important to be alert to such symptoms as nausea, loss of appetite, diarrhea, or visual difficulties.

These may be signs that too much digitalis has accumulated in the body. Too much digitalis can lead to even more serious effects on the heart. It can cause severe slowing of the heart rate or serious irregularities of the heartbeat. This is often sensed as a feeling of palpitation or thumps in the chest.

Even a patient who has been taking digitalis for a long time can develop some of these side effects. So if you notice any symptom that has been mentioned or any other new symptoms, don't pass them off lightly. Don't practice self-diagnosis. Call or see your doctor immediately.

For those people who do not obtain sufficient relief with digitalis and a water pill, there is another class of drugs (vasodilators) that may be added. These drugs cause the small arteries of the body to open widely so that the heart can pump blood into them more easily.

SUMMARY

1. The heart and lungs work together to provide the cells of the body with oxygen. The heart is the pump, and the lungs, the ventilator.

2. Without oxygen, the cells of the body cannot live. They need it to consume food for energy.

3. The heart and lungs can provide reserve energy to meet stressful situations such as exercise. This reserve decreases gradually with age. The more we exercise regularly, the more reserve we have.

4. Heart failure is a condition in which the heart cannot pump enough blood to meet the body's need for oxygen.

5. Shortness of breath and accumulation of fluid are the major signs of heart failure.

6. Treatment of heart failure includes avoiding salt and using water pills to eliminate fluid and digitalis to strengthen the heart.

4

SHORT-WINDEDNESS II:
THE LUNGS
AS THE CULPRIT

Not long ago it was common belief that every cold would
turn into "galloping" pneumonia. We all remember how our
parents practiced the traditional medical rites for driving
out illness, using suffocating vaporizers and sticky chest
rubs. The memory of the pungent scent of eucalyptus lingers
like a musty odor in a damp cellar, reminding us of all those
endless childhood respiratory illnesses. It makes us wonder
why we don't seem to bounce back from a respiratory ailment as quickly as we did when we were children. Do our
lungs fail us as we grow older? The answer is decidedly *no*.
In fact, our breathing strength holds up quite well as the
years pass. True, we do pant a little more than we used to
after exercise, but we can still function at a high level if we
stay in condition. Not all of the problems with breathing can
be blamed directly on our lungs. A heart condition, for example, is often to blame (see page 45). In this chapter we
shall be dealing solely with breathing difficulty caused by
lung problems.

ASTHMA

When it comes to diagnosing asthma, everyone thinks he's a doctor. After all, when you have seen someone with an attack of asthma, you are not likely to forget it. The terrible distress of the person with asthma struggling to inhale and exhale and the musical wheezing sounds he makes leave a lasting impression.

Unfortunately, not everything that resembles asthma is really asthma. This is especially true in older people. Usually the older asthma sufferer has known he has had the condition for many years, but asthma that begins later in life can be confused with many other conditions. This is especially true for heart failure, which can easily be mistaken for asthma (see page 45). Emphysema (see page 62) may masquerade as asthma, and it may require sophisticated breathing tests to distinguish the two.

What exactly is asthma? You will recall that the air we breathe travels in our lungs through progressively smaller branching tubes called *bronchi*, which fan out in both lungs ending finally in countless tiny air sacs, huddled at the very ends like grapes clustered on the vine. The bronchi are flexible tubes able to change their size to regulate the flow of air. During an attack of asthma, these airways contract, their lining begins to swell, and sticky mucus rapidly accumulates. The net effect of all these changes is interference with the flow of air in and out of the lungs. If you have ever choked after inhaling a cloud of smoke, you have some idea of the sense of suffocation a person experiences during an attack of asthma. In the majority of cases of asthma, it is not possible to identify a specific cause, although every effort should be made to do so. Sometimes it turns out to be an allergic reaction to something commonly overlooked in the house, such as feather pillows, fur-bearing animals, or materials used at work. Some people find their attack is triggered by exposure to cold air or even by exercise. More often than not, however, nothing definite can be pinpointed.

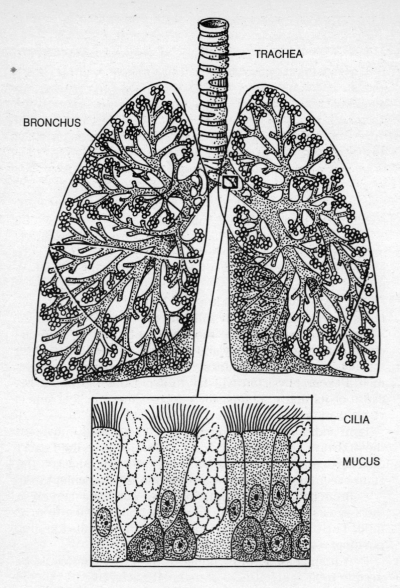

Fig. 13 Mucus surface of bronchus. Normal lungs with the windpipe
(trachea) and branching bronchial tubes and air sacs (alveoli).
Below is a magnified view of the cells lining the bronchial tubes.

TREATMENT OF ASTHMA

There are several classes of medicine used for this purpose:

1. The first line of defense is usually the group of drugs called bronchodilators, which keep the bronchial tubes open by relaxing their muscles. Aminophylline is the most widely used drug of this type.

2. If additional therapy is needed, your physician may add a drug in the adrenaline family that will also open the bronchial tubes. Since that can also cause nervousness and rapid heartbeat, it must be used with caution in older people. A new member of this group, terbutaline, has very little effect on the heart and is the safest one to use.

3. For severe cases due to allergy, chromolyn sodium, which is inhaled as a powder, is very effective. It actually prevents the allergic reaction from affecting the bronchial tubes.

4. Cortisone inhalers are also helpful in preventing attacks in selected people. By inhaling the cortisone, you bring it directly to the bronchial tubes without allowing it to circulate throughout the body and cause side effects.

Occasionally, asthmatics may need to take cortisone by mouth. Your physician will try to avoid this treatment because of its many serious side effects. Close medical supervision is mandatory.

In addition to taking medicine, the asthmatic individual must always remember to drink a great deal of fluid every day, particularly in hot weather. Fluid prevents your sputum from becoming sticky and thus clogging the bronchial tubes.

Bronchodilators, terbutaline, and cortisone are given intravenously in severe attacks along with large quantities of fluid. The usual intravenous bronchodilator is called aminophylline.

It is impossible to mention all the drugs that could be used to treat acute attacks of asthma. Each must be tailored to obtain maximum benefit for the individual, without producing uncomfortable or dangerous side effects. You may require one or several of these medications depending on the nature of your problem.

In one way it is unfortunate that commercial preparations for asthma and chest congestion are so readily accessible. Because of intensive advertising of these products, with dramatic re-creations of people with respiratory distress obtaining instant relief, an older person experiencing similar distress is likely to conclude that his problem must also be asthma. This can lead to serious consequences if his distress is caused by heart trouble, since most asthma preparations have a harmful effect in such cases. So avoid taking any commercial medicines if you develop sudden shortness of breath. These medicines have their place, but until your doctor determines what your problem is, keep away from them.

LUNG DEFENSES

The air we breathe is a vast, invisible ocean teeming with unseen particles. Run your fingers along your windowsill and you'll appreciate the quantities of dust and soot that enter your lungs daily. Why aren't the tiny air chambers of our lungs flooded and eventually clogged by all this floating debris? Despite their microscopic size, these particles become trapped in the tiny air passages before they ever reach the distant air chambers. The first line of defense against this invading cloud of pollutants is the sensitive lining of our air passages, which seizes the soot particles from the flowing current of air by means of a sticky coating called mucus, which behaves somewhat like flypaper. Underneath this sticky film is a carpet of specialized cells that make up most of the inner lining of the bronchial passages. Sprouting from each cell is a dense growth of hairlike projections called *cilia* (see Fig. 13). When millions of these cells are viewed as tightly knit carpet pile, the swaying of their surface hairs resembles a wind swept field of wheat. The gentle swaying rhythm of these protective bristles sweeps the thin mucus coating with its ensnared soot particles upward toward the mouth where they are swallowed or expectorated. Not only soot particles but microorganisms and other dangerous elements in the air we breathe (such as pollen) are trapped within the sticky coating and prevented from reaching the delicate air chambers. We are rarely aware of this defensive action of our lungs. In unusual circumstances, such as sudden smoke inhalation, we may notice a large amount of mucus when we cough.

WHAT IS BRONCHITIS?

Now that you know about some of the protective measures that defend our lungs against harmful substances in the environment, it is easy to understand what we mean by the condition called *bronchitis*. The term *bronchitis* literally means inflammation of the bronchi or air passages. If an invading organism should, for some reason, gain a foothold in the lining of the bronchi, it can irritate and injure the delicate lining cells and temporarily paralyze the sweeping columns of hairs, preventing their cleansing action. With these cleansing hairs out of action, further injury follows. Irritated cells begin to discharge increasing amounts of mucus in response to the spreading infection. While this is happening, the person begins to cough and may develop fever. At first, the amount of mucus coughed up may be scanty and grayish in color, but with worsening infection it increases in amount and becomes thick and yellow. During the peak of the infection, vague burning sensations or tight feelings in the chest and shortness of breath are quite common.

The term *acute bronchitis* is used when an attack occurs in someone without any previous lung condition. Acute bronchitis is apt to occur during the winter months, often in conjunction with outbreaks of flu. Generally the attack subsides within a week or two, although a troublesome dry cough may persist for a somewhat longer period. Older people may find that they can't shake the infection as well as their younger friends or relatives, many of whom have acquired the infection at about the same time. Since a virus is frequently responsible, it is often possible to identify the person who was the source of the infection.

TREATMENT OF ACUTE BRONCHITIS

For the most part treatment is quite simple. Rest is important, but don't use this as an excuse for staying in bed. Avoid going outdoors in the cold until the worst phase of illness has passed. Be sure to take large amounts of fluids, such as juices. Fluids help keep the sputum thin and make it easier to cough it up. Coughing keeps the air passages clear of thick mucus that can cause blockage. So keep away from medicines that eliminate coughing altogether, especially if you have a large amount of mucus. Instead take glyceryl guaicolate, which is a cough medicine that primarily acts to loosen the mucus without preventing coughing. You can usually purchase it at the drugstore. Just as importantly, don't take any commercial preparations that dry out the sputum. These can make the mucus thick like jelly causing blockage of the air passages. You may believe you are improving when the medicine cuts down on the amount of sputum, but in reality this can worsen your breathing problem.

Above all, if you notice large amounts of yellow sputum, high fever, or shortness of breath, see your doctor. You may need antibiotics if the viral infection has led to a bacterial inflammation. Moreover, what seems to be bronchitis to you may actually be a case of pneumonia.

CHRONIC BRONCHITIS

Some people seem to develop frequent attacks of bronchitis over the years. Between attacks, they may have a constant cough and bring up small amounts of phlegm. When this occurs, the condition is called *chronic bronchitis*. In effect there is a persistent, mild inflammation of the bronchial lining. This simmering inflammation undermines the first line of defense of our lungs, the cleansing hairs of the bronchial lining. With this defense line breached, it is easier for microorganisms to gain a foothold leading to new infections.

The person with chronic bronchitis usually knows that a new infection has developed when his sputum increases in amount or changes in color. Very often there will be fever at the time of a new infection.

People who are heavy cigarette smokers (usually over a pack per day) are most prone to develop chronic bronchitis. Chronic bronchitis can eventually lead to severe lung damage and emphysema, which we shall discuss later in the chapter. Not everyone with chronic bronchitis has been a smoker, however. Exposure to severe environmental pollution can also be a major factor. In other instances, poor body resistance and frequent attacks of acute bronchitis can lead to permanent injury to the bronchial tree.

Still, the largest number of people with chronic bronchitis can be found in the ranks of long-term heavy smokers. You'll recognize them easily by the hacking cough that punctuates their every conversation. For these people, the only successful treatment is to stop smoking. The lung has remarkable recuperative powers. People frustrated by the "smoker's cough" that always seems to erupt at the most inopportune time are pleasantly surprised when this source of embarrassment disappears after they stop smoking. This is not to say that no lasting damage remains. But their breathing will usually improve although it may not return to normal.

TREATMENT OF CHRONIC BRONCHITIS

Stop smoking. That's the most important part of the treatment for chronic bronchitis. Once you've done this, there is not much difference in treatment between acute and chronic bronchitis. The attacks of acute infection that frequently interrupt the steady course of the chronic condition should be treated promptly with antibiotics since a bacterial infection is usually responsible in these cases. Certain medications that open up the bronchial passages by reducing the spasm provoked by inflammation can offer some relief both in cases of acute and chronic bronchitis. The most valuable of these types of medication is aminophylline or one of its derivatives. This type of medication can be taken in pill or liquid form. It has proved to be particularly worthwhile when wheezing and shortness of breath accompany the attack.

In all types of bronchitis, it is essential to keep the sputum as thin as possible. The most convenient way of achieving this is by drinking lots of fluid. There are certain types of medication that can play a secondary role but are no more effective than adequate fluid intake. For those who find their sputum so thick that it is difficult to cough up, a steam vaporizer or a room humidifier can be an effective aid.

PRECAUTIONS FOR THE PERSON WITH CHRONIC BRONCHITIS

Since a weakened lung is particularly susceptible to infection, the person with chronic bronchitis must make special efforts to avoid situations likely to lead to infection. For the most part, this simply means using a little common sense:

1. Dress appropriately for the weather.
2. Avoid going outdoors in inclement weather.

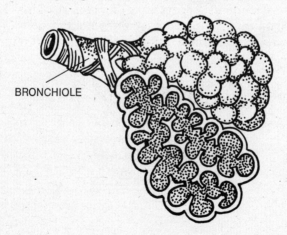

BRONCHIOLE

Fig. 14   Normal alveoli.

3. Postpone visits to friends or relatives who are suffering from viral illnesses.
4. If a new infection develops, have it treated promptly.
5. Get a yearly flu shot. This may give you some protection before outbreaks of flu.

A word here about vitamin C. By now just about everyone has heard of the reputed value of massive doses of vitamin C in preventing colds. While this obviously appeals to everyone's desire for instant health, there is no accepted scientific basis for taking doses of vitamin C that far exceed the body's daily requirement. Some authorities believe that the long-term use of such large quantities of vitamin C may actually be harmful. Such doses probably won't harm most people, but they don't do much good either.

EMPHYSEMA

The term *emphysema* has become popular shorthand for virtually any type of lung problem. But, in fact, emphysema is a very specific type of lung condition.

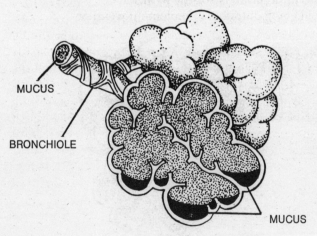

MUCUS

BRONCHIOLE

MUCUS

Fig. 15   Alveoli in emphysema. Note the enlargement and fusion of air sacs.

In emphysema there is injury to the many tiny air chambers that provide our body with oxygen. Normally, as we inhale and exhale, these millions of tiny chambers inflate and collapse together. As emphysema develops, many of these tiny chambers begin to overexpand and rupture; they lose their ability to snap back and deflate, much as a balloon becomes flabby from too frequent use. Normally, the elastic resilience of the air chambers empties them of the carbon dioxide from the blood as we exhale. As these chambers enlarge and become limp in emphysema, air begins to stagnate. Since carbon dioxide cannot be completely expelled, it accumulates in the tiny chambers and therefore in the blood.

Because the air chambers lose some of their flexibility, it becomes increasingly difficult for the person with emphysema to empty his lungs completely and allow fresh air to enter. This leads to lack of oxygen in the blood.

At first glance, the chest of a patient with emphysema seems too well developed for someone with breathing difficulty. On closer inspection, however, it becomes clear that his chest is really disproportionately large for the rest of the body and he must struggle to move air in and out of his lungs. So his chest becomes "barrel shaped" and overinflated as inside his lungs millions of air chambers expand and enlarge. This is emphysema in its worst form. Fortunately, most people never reach this stage. Theirs is much milder with only minimal shortness of breath. Emphysema usually develops over a long period of time but may never reach the point where it is seriously debilitating.

Although there are a number of known causes for emphysema (and in some people no cause is ever found), it turns out that most people with serious emphysema have been long-time heavy smokers. Occasionally, people whose occupations result in continuous exposure to heavy concentrations of certain dust particles like coal, asbestos, or cotton may develop emphysema.

A "TOUCH" OF EMPHYSEMA

Not uncommonly, some older people who notice that a day's exercise makes them puff a little more than they did when they were younger are often told that they have a "touch of emphysema." Just as your skin loses some of its flexible tone, so do other tissues of your body including your lungs. The small loss of elasticity in the air chambers is of no consequence and never leads to any problems. This condition is called *senile emphysema*, a poor choice of words for something as innocent as a few gray hairs. But doctors sometimes use disagreeable terms to describe ordinary problems. So if you've been told you have a "touch of emphysema" and have not been a smoker, just forget about it. If your doctor deems it important, a breathing test will settle the issue. Even if you have been a smoker, the chances are that a slight amount of emphysema will never develop into anything to worry about.

TREATMENT OF EMPHYSEMA

The extent of injury to your lungs will determine in large measure how much difficulty you will have in breathing. While you cannot repair damaged or ruptured air chambers in your lungs, you can help yourself by avoiding further damage to your lungs and participating in a program to improve their efficiency. Here are a few suggestions:

1. Try to avoid the common situations that lead to infections. More than anything else, recurrent lung infections sap the breathing power of people with emphysema. Keep away from crowds during flu epidemics and discourage visits by friends or relatives with colds.

2. Dress appropriately for the weather. If it's not necessary for you to go out on a cold, snowy day or when it's raining, be sensible and stay indoors.

3. Take the yearly flu shot and the newer pneumococcal vaccine. Any treatment that offers some protection against infection is useful.

4. Moving from an area you have lived in for many years is difficult. Yet if long, bitter winters are hurting your breathing more each year, think about moving to where you'll be more comfortable. This also holds true for areas of high pollution. Of course, it isn't easy to begin anew elsewhere, especially when there is no guarantee that it will

bring you improved vitality or well-being. So don't make a hasty decision by yourself. Discuss it carefully with your doctor and family. Try to test the water by an extended visit to the area of your choice to see if you really do experience fewer breathing problems. If not, you haven't lost anything.

5. In hot, humid weather, stay in an air-conditioned environment, but be sure it isn't too cold.

6. Drink substantial quantities of fluids regularly every day, such as juices, especially during hot weather when loss of body water leads to thickened sputum and clogging of the bronchial passages.

7. See your doctor at the first sign of infection such as fever, increased cough, or change in the color of your sputum.

8. There are many types of complicated breathing devices available to assist people with serious breathing problems. It is beyond the scope of this book to discuss when and how they are to be used. Your doctor can advise you about the advantages of these devices, or he may refer you to a specialist in respiratory diseases.

9. Certain types of breathing exercises can strengthen your abdominal muscles to help you breathe easier and better. Your doctor will decide whether these may be of value to you.

10. A few people can benefit from continuous breathing of a steady stream of pure oxygen through a small nasal tube. Portable machines are now available that can be used during routine chores. This type of therapy can be undertaken only under strict medical supervision, since it requires intimate knowledge of the individual respiratory problem. Dire consequences can result from indiscriminate or inappropriate use of such a technique. It goes without saying that no one should take it upon himself to begin such a program on his own. Leave the decision as to whether you are a candidate for this to your doctor or to the specialist he selects.

11. And finally, most importantly, *stop smoking*. No amount of treatment or therapy can be successful if you continue to smoke. Continued smoking simply means more and more injury to your lungs. There's no way around it.

Don't fool yourself by saying you "don't inhale the smoke." There is no way to prevent the poisonous smoke from entering your lungs unless you stop smoking or stop breathing!

BREATHING TESTS

Some people are confused and even frightened by the imposing machines that specialists use to measure breathing performance in patients with lung problems. Actually, the tests are quite simple. They require you to do nothing more than forcefully blow into a tube. The machines do the rest. They provide a great deal of information about the overall efficiency and capacity of your lungs. Expert interpretation of this information can indicate the precise nature of your breathing difficulty and, just as importantly, provide objec-

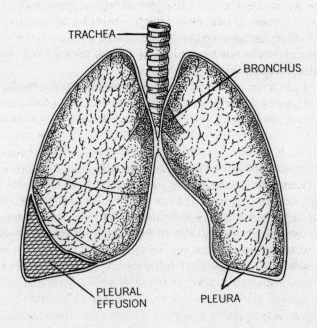

Fig. 16   Diagram of the lungs demonstrating the space between the two pleural layers which cover the lungs and separate them from the chest wall. Note the fluid which has accumulated in the right pleural space.

tive data for assessing your response to treatment and determining progress over a long period of time. So don't be surprised if the tests have to be repeated from time to time.

PLEURISY

A thin sheath (pleura) covers both lungs and adheres as tightly to their surfaces as the rind does to the fruit. A similar lining covers the inner surface of our chest cage that houses the lungs (fig. 16). Inflammation of these coverings is called *pleurisy*. As our lungs expand when we inhale, the two surfaces slide easily against one another. Inflammation roughens the two pleural surfaces so that during breathing they scrape against each other like two sheets of sandpaper. This scraping action produces a sharp, knifelike pain when we take a deep breath. Doctors refer to this type as *pleuritic*. When they listen with a stethoscope, they hear a raspy sound called a *friction rub*.

Many types of injury can lead to inflammation of the pleural surfaces. The resulting pain can be quite severe, making it difficult to take a deep breath without flinching. Yet the condition may not be as serious as it seems. For example, a viral infection of the surface of the lung can cause severe pain, yet in most cases it is a minor condition. This is not meant to imply that pleurisy should be taken lightly. On the contrary, many conditions that cause pleuritic pain may require immediate attention. These include blood clots to the lung, lung tumors, and even serious infections of the pleura. Since it may be risky to wait to see if the pain subsides, the sudden appearance of pleuritic pain is reason enough to see your doctor promptly.

WATER ON THE LUNG

When fluid begins to seep into the space between the two layers of pleura, the condition is called *pleural effusion* or more commonly *water on the lung* (See Fig. 16). The fluid itself does not cause any problems unless very large amounts accumulate, in which case it can interfere with breathing. It is very important to determine why the fluid accumulated in the first place. Very often fluid develops as a result of heart failure (see page 45) and clears up with treatment of this condition. Fluid caused by a viral infection will recede as the infection clears. Unfortunately, sometimes the pleural effusion indicates the presence of a more serious condition such as a tumor. This explains the occasional urgency your doctor expresses in finding the cause of water on the lungs. One of the simplest means for doing this is to examine the fluid after withdrawing a small sample with a needle. The procedure is painless and takes only a minute or two.

Most cases of water on the lung either clear up by themselves or can be successfully treated with medication. Only when breathing is impaired by large collections of fluid will it become necessary to remove significant amounts.

Many cases of water on the lung are due to a relatively straightforward problem. So don't be alarmed if you are told you have water on your lung. Follow your doctor's recommendation and, above all, don't panic if he suggests it is necessary to remove some fluid from your lung.

COUGHING UP BLOOD

The sight of blood frightens many people, more so when it is their own. This is especially true when they cough up blood. Unlike a pain or ache, it's hard to ignore. Yet this is exactly what many people try to do. The most sensible thing to do is see your doctor immediately rather than ignore it or worry. Actually, most of the time there is a simple explanation, such as bronchitis or minor injury to the air passages caused by vigorous coughing. But sometimes a serious problem does exist. If it isn't diagnosed and treated early, it could easily get out of hand. This includes blood clots to the lung, heart failure, and even tuberculosis or other lung infections. Even lung tumors, which people, with good reason, fear the most, can be treated if caught in their early stage.

WHAT WILL THE DOCTOR DO?

First of all, he'll examine you carefully. He may be able to tell what's wrong immediately. Chances are, however, that he'll want a chest X-ray. This is a routine matter and not a sign that he suspects the worst. Some conditions require a more thorough examination of the air passages. To be absolutely certain that nothing serious has been overlooked, your doctor is likely to recommend bronchoscopy. This is a relatively simple test that permits a direct view of the upper air passages using a thin flexible tube. A number of conditions can be promptly diagnosed with this method. It is the most precise means of examining someone who has been coughing up blood.

SPOT ON THE LUNG

The term *spot* or *shadow* on the lung is used to describe any blemish on the usually clear appearance of an X-ray of the lungs. Like many other situations in medicine, this spot can be just a harmless remainder of some long-forgotten lung infection or it may be an early sign of an emerging problem. The discovery of a lung shadow calls for a thorough examination. An old X-ray can be invaluable if it shows that the identical spot was present years before. So if it is possible to obtain some previous X-rays, this can save a great deal of time and effort. In general, bronchoscopy will be required if the shadow is new or appears to be changing, and certainly when someone has been coughing up blood. To dispel any doubt, it will also be necessary to obtain a biopsy. With today's methods, this can often be accomplished without difficulty through the bronchoscope. Unfortunately, it is not always possible to obtain a biopsy without an operation. If it is concluded that the spot is too risky to be left alone, surgery may be suggested.

The presence of a spot on the lung does not necessarily mean that you have a serious problem. But it makes sense to do everything possible to find out exactly what that spot means.

LUNG CANCER

It is almost impossible to pass over some signs of lung cancer such as coughing up blood or an attack of pneumonia. Others, like weakness or weight loss, come on so unobtrusively that it is easy to ignore them or put them out of your mind. A heavy smoker cannot afford to ignore any symptom. Cancer of the lung is the most common internal cancer of men today and it is rising at an alarming rate in women. Everyone knows the dangers of smoking. Its close links to lung cancer and most forms of chronic lung disease have been widely publicized. Yet people continue to smoke even as the pack of cigarettes in their hands warns them that smoking is dangerous to their health.

We have all heard the rationalization, spoken in almost fatalistic resignation, that the "damage has been done anyway." It is naive and foolish to justify smoking with this argument. Injury only grows as the smoking continues. Furthermore, there is a brighter side to the picture. For when you stop smoking, there is an immediate drop in your chances of developing cancer. This risk declines each year thereafter, until the former smoker has no more chance of developing lung cancer than the person who never smoked. The message is clear: *Stop smoking and give your lungs a chance.*

PNEUMONIA

A generation of medical progress has radically changed our perception of pneumonia. There was a time when pneumonia was the sudden draft that snuffed out life in the feeble and, too often, even in the healthy. Though modern drugs have drastically reduced the death toll from pneumonia, we should not lightly dismiss it as a harmless condition. Indeed, in older people, pneumonia can be a very serious and life-threatening matter.

Pneumonia is an inflammation of a number of clustered air chambers in the lung. Many kinds of microorganisms can start this inflammation, but the ultimate effect is the entry of pus cells and fluid into these delicate air chambers (alveoli). It is not completely clear exactly how the invading micro-organism gains its foothold and starts the chain of events leading to pneumonia. It does seem, however, that as we grow older we become more vulnerable to these micro-organisms.

Even more important, in older people it is often hard to make an early diagnosis and the illness tends to be more serious. Typically, a person with pneumonia will experience fever, sweating, coughing with variable amounts of sputum, and shortness of breath. In some older people, however, these symptoms tend to be less striking, or even absent. There may not even be any suggestion of a lung problem. Instead deceptive symptoms may first appear as listlessness, change in behavior, and sudden loss of interest in one's surroundings. Close relatives or friends can usually recognize the sudden change in the person, but if they have not kept close contact, they can easily dismiss the slowness of thought and loss of interest as just another sign of age.

This common reaction illustrates the need for society to rid itself of outmoded stereotypes of how older people behave. Peculiar behavior that would arouse immediate concern in a younger person is often ignored in older people simply because it is expected of them. Too often this leads to needless delay in getting to the doctor and having the illness diagnosed. Prolonged suffering could be prevented by early treatment.

Medical attention is often delayed not only for pneumonia but for a variety of other conditions that cause odd behavior in older people. Past generations of doctors stood by helplessly, watching the vitality ebb in pneumonia patients. Today all this has changed. Most people, no matter what their age, will recover from pneumonia.

TYPES OF PNEUMONIA

A variety of microorganisms can cause pneumonia. The most common of these are viruses or bacteria. Bacterial infections can be treated with antibiotics. For the viral pneumonias, we do not have any effective treatment. When your doctor is not sure whether your pneumonia is caused by viruses or bacteria, he may play it safe and prescribe an antibiotic for you.

Generally, we rely on our body's natural defenses to deal with viral infections. But, sometimes in the struggle against this kind of infection, the body's defenses may be weakened and then a bacterial infection will gain a foothold. If this happens, it will then become necessary to give the person antibiotics.

Antibiotics are not necessary for every chest infection. Your doctor will decide whether you have a simple viral infection that will clear up by itself or whether you need antibiotic treatment. Don't diagnose yourself. Don't use someone else's antibiotics or some pills left on the shelf. Used incorrectly, these drugs can do more harm than good.

LEGIONNAIRE'S DISEASE

In recent years an unusual type of pneumonia that seems to have eluded medical scientists until now has captured headlines. Because an American Legion Convention was the scene of its first deadly and dramatic appearance, it has been called Legionnaire's disease. Afterward, scientists were able to show that this disease is caused by a peculiar strain of bacteria that is very difficult to identify. It seems to grow wherever there is stagnant water, such as in the cooling towers of central air-conditioning systems. This explains summertime epidemics in areas of large businesses or hotels.

During this first outbreak, a large number of people succumbed to the infection. Since then, its mere mention creates panic. Public Health authorities must assume some of the blame for this type of reaction since their highly publicized crusades whenever a few cases surface feed people's fears. In all likelihood, this illness has been with us for years, masquerading as "flu" or another respiratory illness. While it remains a serious infection, Legionnaire's disease will probably prove to be less fearsome than its current reputation. Like most bacterial infections, the disease responds to antibiotic treatment. The antibiotic of choice is called erythro-mycin.

Since older people and people with chronic illness fare worse when the disease strikes, they should be especially aware of its symptoms and get prompt treatment. As a rule, the disease begins with weakness and a generally sick feeling. High fever with chills develops rapidly together with frequent chest pain and diarrhea. You don't have to be afraid of catching Legionnaire's disease from someone else. It does not appear to be transmitted from person to person.

SUMMARY

1. Not all shortness of breath is caused by lung problems. Do not diagnose yourself. Find out from your doctor whether this is your problem.

2. Shortness of breath and wheezing may look like asthma, but this is not always so. Never use commercial medications without first consulting your doctor.

3. Nowhere is it more obvious than with regard to respiratory infections that "an ounce of prevention is worth a pound of cure." Just practice simple common sense in dress habits, cut down exposure to cold, and avoid people with respiratory infections.

4. Coughing up blood may be due to an innocent condition. But don't take any chances. See your doctor at once and put your fears to rest.

5. Pneumonia is treatable but it comes in many disguises. Any unusual behavior in an older person should be viewed with suspicion whether or not a cough is present.

6. The person who doesn't smoke is unlikely to develop chronic bronchitis or emphysema. In addition, he has a much lower risk of cancer of the lung. If you stop smoking, you will decrease your risks.

5

VARICOSE VEINS: GUILT BY ASSOCIATION

As we get older, most of us, at one time or another, worry about the veins of our legs, how they look, what trouble they may cause or are causing us. Much has been written and said about these veins; much of it useful and sound and helpful. But, at the same time, much misinformation has gotten abroad, too, and has caused undue anxiety to patients and in some cases, unnecessary and dangerous therapies or "cures."

In what follows, we shall be setting forth the facts about vein problems (varicose veins and blood clots). In particular, we shall be pointing out why varicose veins are not dangerous and usually require no treatment at all.

HOW VEINS WORK

The role of the veins is to carry blood back to the heart after it has delivered oxygen and nutrients to the cells of the body and picked up waste products. If you look at the underside of your forearm, you can see thin blue streaks under your skin. These are veins. They are blue because they have very little oxygen in them.

74

The manner in which veins carry out their function is quite intricate. When you stand up, the veins must find a way of getting the blood in the legs to move against gravity back to the heart. Since they have no muscles, they cannot accomplish this alone. It is the muscles in our limbs that must help move the blood. As we walk, the muscles of our legs squeeze against the veins and cause the blood to move. On the other hand, if we stand or even lie still, a great deal of blood remains motionless in the leg veins.

What determines the direction of blood flow? If the veins were only tubes filled with blood, squeezing them would force blood to move haphazardly in all directions. The unique mechanism in the veins that makes the blood flow in the right direction is a series of delicate one-way valves that allow the blood to travel in only one direction: toward the heart. These valves are part of the inside wall of each vein and open only in the direction of the heart (fig. 17).

There are two sets of veins in the legs; superficial veins that are visible just under the skin and deep veins lying under the muscles. Under normal conditions, most of the blood is carried toward the heart by the deep veins, which we cannot see.

DEEP-VEIN CLOTS: DIAGNOSIS

The major problm with deep veins arises out of the formation of clots. A clot (*thrombosis*) in a vein is variously called *thrombophlebitis*, *phlebitis*, or *venous thrombosis*. These clots can vary in length from inches to several feet.

The dangers of such clotting are twofold: 1) The valves of the veins may be permanently damaged. 2) A piece of the clot may break off from the main portion of clot and travel to the lungs (*plumonary embolus*). More about these serious complications later (see page 80).

Blood clots form mostly in sedentary people who do not exercise regularly or move the muscles of their legs. They, therefore, cannot pump the blood toward the heart. Even when we sit for hours at a time, the small, aimless move-

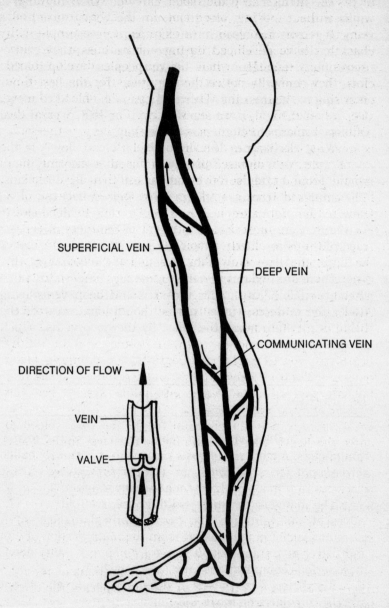

SUPERFICIAL VEIN

DEEP VEIN

COMMUNICATING VEIN

DIRECTION OF FLOW

VEIN

VALVE

Fig. 17 Veins of the leg. Insert shows valve which allows flow of blood in only one direction (toward the heart).

ments of our legs keep the blood moving. When, however, we sit without moving, blood clots are likely to form in our veins. It is not uncommon, for example, to see people with clots that have developed during a long bus or car ride. Interestingly enough, when active people develop blood clots, they generally notice the symptoms for the first time on arising in the morning. Their clots usually develop during sleep when their legs are least active. For this reason, the restless sleeper, although he or she may be a bothersome bedmate, is less likely to develop these clots.

People with diseases or conditions that prevent their moving around often suffer blood clots in their legs. Thus, a limb paralyzed from a stroke or immobilized because of a fractured hip, for example, is extremely prone to blood clots. For this reason, most doctors advise early surgery to repair fractured hips in elderly people. The sooner they can move the limb, the less likely they are to have blood clots. In general, doctors today try not to prescribe bedrest for prolonged periods because clots may form within a few days. After surgery, doctors usually want their patients out of bed within twenty-four hours.

Blood clots tend to form in people with unhealthy hearts. If, for example, the heart is not pumping blood quickly enough into the arteries and capillaries (heart failure, see page 45), the whole circulatory system becomes backed up. Too much blood is left behind in the veins because there is not enough room for all the veins' blood to enter the heart. Blood remaining in the legs, under these conditions, cannot move and so it often clots. The problem in heart failure is really analogous to rush-hour traffic in which lack of forward motion of the front cars leads to a bumper-to-bumper line of cars behind them.

When clotting takes place in a deep vein (phlebitis), the leg swells rapidly, usually within hours or at most a couple of days. The swelling is greatest at the ankle, and becomes progressively less in the upper portions of the leg. There may be pain in the calf or the inner part of the thigh. Sometimes the leg may feel warm.

Unfortunately, many people incorrectly ascribe all kinds of symptoms to phlebitis. They have read about blood clots and are afraid that they will have circulation problems or clots in their lungs. In 1974, the public's fear of phlebitis reached epidemic proportions when Richard Nixon developed serious, life-threatening blood clots.

To make matters worse, many physicians tend to attribute pain in the leg to phlebitis when they can't find another cause. This leads to frequent misdiagnosis and to wrong and dangerous treatment. These mistakes would not occur if doctors remembered the importance of swelling of the leg for the diagnosis of phlebitis. Swelling without pain is often phlebitis, but pain without swelling is almost never phlebitis.

DEEP-VEIN CLOTS: TREATMENT

Once clots form in the deep veins of the legs, they must be treated quickly. Untreated, they may continue to move up the leg and cause inflammation in the wall of the vein. As the clot extends, the inflammation in the wall of the vein also spreads upward. The inflammation may involve the vein's delicate valves and leave them scarred. As a result, these valves no longer function properly and there is no way to control the direction of blood flow. Blood then tends to accumulate in the veins of the leg. For this reason, a leg that has had phlebitis once is always more susceptible to another attack. If enough valves are damaged, there may be permanent damage to the circulation in the leg. Similarly, the longer the clot becomes, the more likely it is that a piece will break off and travel to the lungs.

If your doctor finds that you have deep-vein phlebitis, he will hospitalize you and generally begin treatment with an anticoagulant (anticlotting) medicine. This medicine will not dissolve the clot that has already formed, but it will prevent it from extending up the vein toward the heart and lungs. Heparin is usually the first drug given and it is usually very effective. Given by injection into a vein, heparin makes it more difficult for blood to clot. Your blood must be carefully tested each day to make sure the dose is just right. Too little heparin would not be effective, and too much heparin might cause bleeding from any area of the body.

Since heparin does not dissolve the clot that is already present, the symptoms of phlebitis will take some time to go away. Much of the initial swelling and tenderness will be gone within a few days, but some swelling will linger on for a few weeks. The clot is gradually dissolved by the body's own system through a series of chemical reactions in the blood. This process usually takes from six to eight weeks. So, after a few days in bed, the swelling may completely subside but reappear when you are on your feet again. Expect this to happen if you have phlebitis and you will spare yourself a great deal of needless alarm and anxiety. This swelling tends to subside at night when you are asleep. It increases gradually during the day when you are up and about. Don't worry. This is part of the normal recovery process.

After seven to fourteen days of treatment, an anticoagulant pill can be substituted for the heparin injections, and you can go home as soon as the doctor has decided on the right dose of these pills for you. How long you will need this medicine depends on your chances of contracting phlebitis again. It is advisable for everyone to have at least eight weeks of treatment because the clot is still present during the first eight weeks. If you are sedentary or have heart problems, your physician may want to have you take the anticoagulant pill for several months or, in some cases, even years. You will need to have a blood test performed regularly to make sure you are taking the right dose, weekly at first and later, monthly.

CHRONIC COMPLICATIONS OF DEEP-VEIN CLOTS

If the valves of the veins have been badly damaged from an attack of phlebitis, chronic symptoms may develop. Much of the blood does not move out of the veins, and the weight of the blood strains the leg, especially when you stand up. As a result, the leg gets swollen and sometimes open sores (ulcers) develop around the ankles. The skin around the ankles may become scaly and itchy (*stasis dermatitis*).

It is important to treat these symptoms before severe

swelling, ulceration, and scarring disfigure the leg. If there is persistent swelling after an attack of phlebitis, you should apply some form of elastic support to the leg. This support should fit properly, more snugly at the ankle and less tightly further up the leg. Elastic support can help keep blood going toward the heart as the leg muscles pump.

You can obtain adequate support with the use of elastic bandages if they are properly applied. Your doctor or nurse will show you how to apply the bandage evenly and firmly from the foot to a level above the swelling, either just below the knee or at the mid-thigh region. If you do not want to bother with these bandages, you can buy a measured surgical stocking prescribed by your doctor. The bandages are, of course, much less expensive than the stockings. Elastic supports should be put on when you get out of bed in the morning and removed at bedtime. Your elastic bandage or stocking will lose its elasticity after a few months, and so you must replace it regularly.

If your leg swells every day, avoid standing for a long time, and elevate your leg several times during the day for periods of ten to fifteen minutes. Walking with an elastic support is good for the circulation, but standing still prevents movement of blood. If you notice some swelling of your leg when you awaken in the morning, try to sleep with your foot elevated three to four inches above the level of your head. You can do this by placing three-inch blocks under the feet of your bed or by putting one or two pillows under your feet.

PULMONARY EMBOLISM (BLOOD CLOTS IN THE LUNGS)

The other major and potentially more serious complication of phlebitis is blood clots traveling to the lungs. In this condition, called *pulmonary embolism*, a piece of the clot extending up a vein breaks off, travels to the heart, and is then pumped into one of the arteries going to the lungs (pulmonary artery). The pulmonary arteries are vital to our existence because they transport the blood into the lungs where oxygen is picked up to be delivered throughout the body. If enough of these arteries become blocked, the person will choke to death just as if he were drowning or in an airless room. Giving him oxygen cannot completely overcome the problem because the oxygen cannot reach the bloodstream. The chances of recovery depend on the person's general health and how many pieces of clot have gone to the lungs.

Unfortunately, pulmonary embolism frequently occurs without the warning of phlebitis in the leg. This happens for two reasons. First, most vein clots cause no symptoms because they are in small veins, and the leg does not swell. A piece of this unnoticed clot can break off and go to the lungs without causing leg symptoms. Second, the clot may travel from a vein located in the lower abdomen rather than the leg. Fortunately, the first attack of pulmonary embolism is rarely fatal, and the chances of survival are excellent if treatment is begun immediately.

When a blood clot enters an artery in the lungs, the first thing you will notice is difficulty in breathing that begins rather suddenly. If the clot is a little larger, you may sweat from the strain of breathing and even faint. If the clot is small, you may have only mild breathing difficulty and it will pass quickly. If the clot is large, your lips may turn blue, and you may remain short of breath for several days. Other symptoms of clots in the lung include chest pain when you take a deep breath and coughing up blood.

Even if the breathing difficulty passes quickly, see your doctor as soon as possible. A mild blood clot may be followed by a whole series of larger clots in the lungs. Your physician must examine you and order laboratory tests to determine whether a blood clot is present in the lungs.

DIAGNOSIS AND TREATMENT OF PULMONARY EMBOLISM

One of the most helpful procedures in proving the presence or absence of pulmonary embolism is called a *lung scan*. In this test, a radioactive material injected into a vein travels through the bloodstream to the lungs. A scanning machine moves back and forth over the chest while the patient is lying on a table. This scanner records the radioactivity in the lungs. If there is a clot in one of the lungs' arteries, the radioactive material cannot reach the portion of lung that it serves. The scan then shows a blank area without radioactivity. An even more accurate procedure is called *pulmonary arteriography*. This is an X-ray test that actually shows the blockage in a lung artery.

The treatment of blood clots in the lungs is the same as treatment for phlebitis, with some added measures. Here anticoagulant drugs are used in the same way in order to prevent more clots. Our bodies usually dissolve the lung clots within two to three weeks. To relieve the shortness of breath, it is usually necessary to administer oxygen in the hospital for a few days. If the blood clot has damaged the heart, this condition must be treated with Digitalis to strengthen the heart and water pills to eliminate fluid from the body.

If you have problems with bleeding, your doctor will stop giving you heparin. It may then be necessary to perform an operation to prevent any other blood clots from traveling to the lungs. Since most blood clots come from the legs, he may ask a surgeon to block the main vein coming from the legs (inferior vena cava). This can usually be accomplished by passing a special device shaped like an umbrella through a jugular vein in the neck. The umbrella is manipulated into the inferior vena cava where it blocks the blood flow in this vein. The umbrella remains there permanently and is quite effective in preventing clots from reaching the lungs. This procedure may also be necessary if you have a blood clot while receiving heparin. Occasionally, insertion of the umbrella is not feasible and then the surgeon may find it necessary to tie off this large vein. This involves abdominal surgery.

A new kind of treatment for blood clots in the lungs has just become available. These drugs (streptokinase and urokinase) can actually make the clots disappear by stimulating the body's own chemical system to dissolve them sooner. Sometimes, these clots are completely gone within one to two days when this medication is used. The risk of internal bleeding is greater with these drugs than with the conven-

tional anticoagulant drugs, and so your physician is unlikely to use them except under very special circumstances.
They may be useful for someone who has had many clots
over a short period of time and is in danger of dying. By
opening some of the lungs' arteries rapidly, streptokinase
may save one's life.

PREVENTION OF BLOOD CLOTS

Can phlebitis and blood clots in the lungs be prevented?
To a degree, yes. If you lead a physically active life and keep
the muscles of your legs functioning, you are very unlikely
to suffer from these blood clots. We run into major problems
when we are forced to be inactive. For example, confinement
to bed because of illness or after an operation may cause
blood clots to develop within a few days. This is why doctors
emphasize early walking after an illness or operation. Even
after a major illness like a heart attack, your doctor will try
to get you out of bed as soon as possible. Even while in bed,
you should move your legs frequently rather than lie perfectly still.

The last few years have seen some important advances
in the prevention of blood clots. We now know that we can
give the anticoagulant drug heparin in low doses to prevent
clot formation in the veins of people who have surgery or are
in bed because of a heart attack. It can be injected two or
three times a day in doses so low that there is very little
danger of bleeding. On the basis of a great deal of experience,
many experts in this field now believe that anybody over the
age of forty or fifty undergoing a major operation should
have this low-dose heparin for a few days after surgery. It
certainly seems a wise treatment for people with a previous
history of phlebitis or blood clots. There is also some evidence
that ordinary aspirin can prevent clots by blocking the platelets in the blood from coming together and starting the clotting process. Oddly enough, aspirin seems to work better in
men (see page 99).

SUPERFICIAL PHLEBITIS

Thus far, we have been discussing clots in the deep veins and their complications. There is another kind of phlebitis that involves the superficial veins (*superficial thrombophlebitis*). This disorder appears as an inflamed area on the skin. If you have this kind of phlebitis, you will feel sharp, localized pain and notice a red, tender, hot area that stands out from the normal skin. If you feel it carefully, you will notice a thickened area under the red skin shaped like a rope or cord. This cord is the superficial vein, inflamed and clotted. Unlike deep phlebitis, which may not be tender at all, superficial phlebitis is always painful, tender, and obviously inflamed when it first begins. As it subsides, the pain and tenderness diminish. The cord usually becomes thinner but may not disappear completely.

Superficial phlebitis does not pose the same dangers as deep phlebitis. The clots in superficial veins almost never break off and travel to the lungs. Since most of the blood is normally carried by the deep veins, we do not have to worry about any chronic problems arising from superficial phlebitis. Anticoagulant drugs are usually unnecessary. Treatment consists of rest, warm soaks to the inflamed area, and an anti-inflammatory drug. In mild cases, aspirin suffices. The phlebitis generally subsides in five to ten days. A persistent, non-tender cord or lump represents only the scarred vein and is nothing to worry about.

DANGER OF SUPERFICIAL PHLEBITIS

The only place where superficial phlebitis can be somewhat dangerous is in the upper part of the thigh. If the clot reaches this level, it can proceed upward to the groin, where it will meet the deep vein. If you notice a red, hot streak in this area, you should seek immediate medical attention. Your doctor will want to hospitalize you and treat you with heparin. In fact, if the streak comes very close to the groin, he may ask for a surgical consultation. The surgeon may recommend a simple operation under local anesthesia.

Through a simple incision in the groin, he can tie off the main superficial vein (greater saphenous vein) and prevent the clot from rising any higher.

CAUSES OF SUPERFICIAL PHLEBITIS

Like deep phlebitis, superficial phlebitis occurs mostly when the blood doesn't circulate well. Therefore, it is generally found only in prominent (varicose) veins. If you contract superficial phlebitis in the absence of varicose veins, your doctor will have to perform a number of tests in order to determine the cause. Sometimes, a hidden cancer may be the cause and so a thorough search is necessary.

VARICOSE VEINS: DIAGNOSIS AND TREATMENT

What is a varicose vein? A varicose vein is merely a superficial vein whose valves function poorly. The blood goes backward (away from the heart) when the person stands up. This is why these veins balloon. Varicose veins do not cause swelling of the leg or impair the circulation. Their only complications are superficial phlebitis and occasional bleeding if they are injured. Neither complication is dangerous. The bleeding can be stopped by pressing the finger on the bleeding point and elevating the leg above heart level.

Varicose veins, although very common, are not dangerous. About 20 percent or more of all women over the age of sixty have varicose veins in their legs, but these varicose veins rarely cause any trouble.

Many doctors blame varicose veins for the complications of deep-vein disease such as swelling and ulceration of the legs. These complications are often seen in association with varicose veins but are not caused by varicose veins. Here, the varicose veins are actually the result of damage to the deep veins.

Most patients with varicose veins have no other problems with their legs. These varicose veins are usually the result of the ordinary wear and tear of life. They are more common in women because of the strains of pregnancies.

Many women notice their varicose veins for the first time during pregnancy. Some people inherit superficial veins with weak valves and so they are more likely to get varicose veins.

Surgery is almost never necessary for the treatment of varicose veins. Unfortunately, thousands of unnecessary operations to remove varicose veins (venous stripping operations) are performed every year. This surgery does not eliminate swelling of the leg and does not cure any symptoms. It is done almost always to improve the appearance of the leg. Even then, it is often unsuccessful because the varicosities frequently come back a few years later.

Much more effective than surgery, particularly for older people, is the use of elastic stockings or bandages. These elastic supports will prevent both superficial phlebitis and bleeding. No other treatment is necessary.

SUMMARY

1. Vein problems in the legs are very common, especially in older people.

2. Sudden swelling of the leg usually means that there is a clot in a deep vein.

3. These clots can damage the veins and travel to the lungs.

4. Keeping active is the best way to prevent these clots from forming.

5. If you have chronic swelling of your legs, wear elastic stockings or bandages.

6. Varicose veins are not dangerous. Surgery for them is almost never necessary.

6

UNDERSTANDING HIGH BLOOD PRESSURE AND STROKE

You're going to see your doctor for your periodic checkup. You haven't been having any unusual or new symptoms, just the same assortment of pains and aches that your doctor has been treating quite satisfactorily and that you've learned to live with. Now your doctor examines you and tells you you have high blood pressure. Now, what do you really know about what has happened and what the future will be like for you? Do you know what high blood pressure is, what it means, what your medication is, and what it will do for you, how long you'll have to take it? Do you know how your doctor finds out you have high blood pressure?

Good questions, and important ones. You should have the answers. First, you have now joined a very large "club." Over 20 million Americans have high blood pressure (*hypertension*). You're lucky. You are one of the 10 million who know they have it and are being treated for it. Over 5 million Americans have high blood pressure and don't know it. Another 5 million know they have high blood pressure, but aren't being treated for it. These unlucky, untreated millions, unless they find out what they have and are treated for it, are in great danger of getting heart disease, a stroke, or dying early. Unfortunately, high blood pressure rarely causes symptoms until these complications develop. A few people may have frequent headaches as a warning sign, but most of the time, there is no warning. Obviously then, everyone should have his blood pressure checked once a year.

WHAT IS HIGH BLOOD PRESSURE?

When your doctor takes your blood pressure, he records two numbers with a line between them—for example, 120/80. This means a systolic pressure of 120 and a diastolic pressure of 80. The systolic pressure is the pressure during a heartbeat, and the diastolic pressure is the pressure in between beats. Since the heart is resting more often than beating, diastolic pressure is closer to the average pressure in our arteries and is the more important reading.

There is still some debate over what constitutes a normal blood pressure, but we can draw some rough guidelines. Generally, the second number (diastolic pressure) should not frequently or consistently be over 95. The first number (systolic pressure) varies with age. Under the age of fifty, the systolic pressure should probably not be consistently over 140 to 150 in healthy people. As we get older, we all develop a certain degree of stiffening of our arteries, and the systolic pressure may rise. This should not, however, raise the diastolic pressure.

It is important to remember that one's blood pressure is not always the same. We can obtain quite different blood pressure readings from time to time in almost anyone if we change the conditions under which we check it. For example, exercise raises the systolic pressure because the heart beats harder, but has little effect on the diastolic pressure. The diastolic pressure may even drop during exercise because the arterioles in our muscles open wider. Hardening of the arteries, as we get older, may profoundly raise the systolic pressure because the stiff walls can no longer stretch when the heart beats. Anxiety, tension, and fear can raise both systolic and diastolic pressures by making the heart beat harder and closing down the arterioles.

We decide that someone has high blood pressure only

after we have found that his blood pressure tends to be high most of the time. We can determine this only by checking blood pressure on several occasions. Hypertension should not be diagnosed without first finding an elevated blood pressure (usually systolic and diastolic) on at least three consecutive tests with the individual as relaxed as possible. Unfortunately, some people become so nervous in a doctor's office that their pressure is always recorded as high even if they don't have hypertension. In such cases, home blood pressure measurements by a family member may give a truer picture of the blood pressure.

WHY WORRY ABOUT HIGH BLOOD PRESSURE?

High blood pressure spells trouble. First, it can lead to serious heart disease. As we pointed out earlier, people with high blood pressure stand a greater chance of developing heart attacks and anginal chest pains because the arteries to the heart itself apparently become clogged more easily if the blood pressure remains high.

In addition to leading to heart attacks, high blood pressure damages the heart in another way. With a higher pressure in the large arteries, the heart has to pump harder to make the blood circulate. As a result of this extra work, the heart must enlarge to handle the strain. As the years go by, this strain pushes the heart to a point where it cannot get any larger. The result of this persistent strain is heart failure and backing up of fluid into the lungs (see page 45).

High blood pressure can also affect the kidneys. The little blood vessels in the kidneys are damaged, and the kidneys don't receive enough blood. The result can be serious impairment of kidney function.

High blood pressure has its most dangerous effects on the brain. The brain is the most vulnerable organ in the body. It is easily injured if there is even a very short interruption in the amount of blood it receives. It must have a continuous supply of oxygen, which it uses up very rapidly. High blood pressure causes a hardening of the arteries. When this

happens, the brain doesn't get all the oxygen it needs because
the arteries leading to the brain become clogged or narrow.
The area in the brain fed by the clogged artery dies in the
same way that a piece of heart muscle dies when it is deprived of oxygen. In the heart, we call this a *myocardial
infarction* or heart attack. In the brain, we call it a *cerebro-
vascular accident* or *stroke*.

While high blood pressure is only one of several equally
important causes of heart attacks, it is without question the
most important cause of strokes. The other factors leading to
heart attack, such as diabetes and smoking, also play a role
in causing strokes, but they are not as important as high
blood pressure. The overwhelming majority of people with
strokes have had high blood pressure for a number of years.

STROKES

What happens when someone has a stroke? The symptoms
usually develop suddenly and depend on how much and
what part of the brain is involved. They can vary from un-
consciousness to a mild weakness. Most commonly, a person
having a stroke suddenly notices weakness or paralysis, usually in an arm and/or a leg on the same side of the body.
Generally, there will be a loss of sensation and a sagging of
the face on the same side as the paralysis because of a weakness in the facial muscles. This happens because special
nerve cells in the brain that direct movement and perceive
sensation have been damaged.

The nerve pathways in the brain crisscross before they
reach the spinal cord. So the nerve cells on the right side of
the brain send signals to nerve cells on the left side of the
spinal cord and vice versa. Therefore, a stroke that damages
nerve cells on one side of the brain will produce paralysis of
the limbs and loss of sensation on the other side of the body.

We can explain the other common symptoms of strokes
by noting the differences between the two sides of the brain.
They are not identical. One side of the brain is dominant

because it is responsible for some of the highly specialized functions that human beings can perform, namely, speaking, communication, and integration of thoughts. In all right-handed people and the majority of left-handed people, the left side of the brain is dominant. Only in some left-handed people is the right side dominant. Thus, in most cases, a stroke involving the right side of the brain will usually leave the patient alert and able to communicate vocally and in writing. On the other hand, a stroke on the left side will often lead to serious deficits in speech and communication as well as right-sided paralysis.

These deficits in communication are called *aphasias* and are very complex. In some people, the damage may be mild, involving only a difficulty in expressing the names of objects and people. The patient may recognize a pen, for example, and know how to use it but not be able to call it a pen. In other cases, the individual may not be able to speak coherently or at all. In the most severe cases, a patient may be erroneously thought to be unconscious when he is just unable to receive or transmit any specific information. He is, however, awake and may be aware of his surroundings even though he doesn't talk or follow commands.

Fortunately, most people recover from strokes by themselves within a few days, and many others gradually improve in the following two to three months. Intensive, daily physiotherapy can help this healing process greatly. This therapy should start immediately even if there is complete paralysis of an arm and leg. Muscles become weak very quickly if they are not exercised. Movement of these muscles by the therapist in the early days after a stroke keeps them in shape so that they can function after the brain cells recover.

It is also very important to protect the joints of the arms and legs. If the muscles around the shoulder become too lax, the upper arm bone (humerus) may fall out of its shoulder socket. This dislocation can prevent full use of the arm later even after strength has returned. Thus, if the shoulder sags badly, it may be necessary to put the arm in a sling temporarily. Fingers can become stiff and eventually useless if they remain immobile and bent into a fist. Splinting the paralyzed hand and fingers in an open, unbent position can prevent this complication.

As someone recovers from a stroke, it is important to help him use whatever muscles he can. This aids his recovery because those muscles that can move may assist other muscles. Even after improvement has stopped, it is important to continue some physiotherapy in order to maintain muscular strength and coordination at the highest level possible.

APHASIA

The aphasias are very difficult to treat. Fortunately again, many people overcome their speech problems on their own especially if they have only a mild disability to begin with. Those who have lost only the ability to name some objects often improve quickly. But people with profound speech impairment generally have a difficult time. It is important to provide speech therapy for them if they are alert enough to benefit from it. The more determined and persevering they are, the more likely it is that they will improve with speech therapy.

SMALL STROKES

As with many other medical problems, the dramatic stroke is only the tip of an iceberg. We are also subject to so-called small strokes (transient ischemic attacks). These are much more frequent than the major, obvious strokes and may be forerunners of a major stroke. People with hardening of the arteries to the brain may develop transient symptoms lasting from minutes to hours. These symptoms are often so subtle that they go almost unnoticed. They include:

1. Sudden numbness of an arm, leg or side of the face
2. Clumsiness of a hand
3. Dropping objects easily
4. Walking unsteadily
5. Dragging of a leg

6. Slurring of speech and mispronouncing words
7. Temporary loss of vision in one eye
8. Dizziness
9. Blurred vision
10. Fainting attacks
11. Temporary loss of speech
12. Forgetfulness
13. Loss of concentration
14. Confusion

If you have any of these symptoms on several occasions, it is possible that you are having little strokes even if the symptoms last only a few minutes. You must get to a doctor quickly.

Your doctor will ask for a very detailed description of your symptoms. He will also examine your nerve and muscle function carefully. He may have to check your memory, your ability to think, and your facility with simple arithmetic. He may even ask you obvious questions about current events. You should not be upset by these questions. Your doctor is trying to see whether you have suffered any brain damage. He may want you to consult a neurologist.

Once your doctor suspects the presence of these little strokes, he must find out what is causing them. Hardening of the arteries is the usual underlying cause for the above symptoms, but there are other causes. If they can be avoided, the person can be often spared the little strokes and possibly even the larger strokes. All of these possible causes are discussed in this book.

1. Abnormal changes in heart rhythm that decrease flow of blood (see page 35)
2. Anemia (see page 199)
3. Low blood-sugar level (see page 112)
4. Postural hypotension (fall in blood pressure when you stand up, see page 209)
5. Chronic use of sedatives and tranquilizers (see page 257)

Changes in heart rhythm are often very fleeting, and twenty-four-hour monitoring may be necessary to pick them up (see page 36).

TREATMENT FOR HARDENING OF
THE ARTERIES

If hardening of the brain's arteries is the only cause of your
symptoms, your doctor has two basic approaches available
to him: medical and surgical. A number of drugs have been
tried with mixed results. Some of these drugs (vasodilators)
help small arteries (arterioles) to open up. They have been
used for many years with many reports of patient improvement. But these claims are difficult to judge because small
strokes may stop occurring for no obvious reason. There is
no definite evidence that people taking these vasodilator
drugs do better than those who do not receive them.

Blood-thinning medications (anticoagulants) have also
been used for many years. These are the same medications
that are used to treat phlebitis. Again the results are quite
mixed. Some physicians have reported that patients benefit
greatly from these drugs while others have found them useless. If you are taking anticoagulants, you must always be on
the alert for bleeding anywhere. In addition, you must have
periodic blood tests to make sure that you are taking the
correct dose. People with persistent high blood pressure
cannot take anticoagulants because of the hazard of bleeding within the brain itself.

The newest treatment involves the use of drugs that
block the action of the platelets. You will recall from an
earlier chapter that platelets are cells traveling in the bloodstream that start the clotting of blood. They protect us from
serious bleeding. Without them, we would be in danger of a
life-threatening hemorrhage every time we cut a finger.
However, their presence is a double-edged sword. They also
start the clotting that clogs arteries and thus play a role in
hardening of arteries. Many small strokes seem to be caused
by the clumping of platelets in small brain arteries. If we
can stop the platelets from clumping, perhaps we can avoid
the strokes.

The most famous of these antiplatelet drugs is simple
aspirin. Recent studies have shown that aspirin taken one
tablet four times a day may prevent strokes in men. It ap-

parently has no value in women. Two other agents, dipyridamole and sulfinpyrazone, also block clumping of platelets but in a different way from aspirin. Many doctors now combine aspirin with one of these other agents in an effort to prevent strokes. We won't have conclusive evidence about the usefulness of these drugs for some time.

SURGICAL TREATMENT FOR SMALL STROKES

In some cases, people having small strokes can benefit from surgery aimed at unclogging one or more of the major arteries to the brain. In order to understand what this surgery entails, you must know a little about the anatomy of the arteries supplying blood to the brain. The front of the brain receives its blood mainly from the two *carotid arteries* that run under the skin of the neck, one on each side. The back of the brain receives its blood supply from two *vertebral arteries*, which are branches of the main arteries going to the arms (*subclavian arteries*). There are also communicating arteries that connect the carotid and vertebral systems on the surface of the brain. (See Fig. 1.)

There are several situations in which surgery is possible. If a carotid artery is blocked somewhere in the neck, a surgeon can open it and remove the clots so that blood can flow more easily again. This procedure entails a risk because you can actually have a stroke while this important artery is being manipulated. However, for someone having repeated small strokes, the risk is relatively small compared to the potential benefit. Your physician can suspect a carotid blockage if he feels a weak pulse in the neck or hears a noise over the artery when he applies a stethoscope to the neck. Similarly, a blocked subclavian artery, which can reduce flow to the vertebral arteries, can be repaired.

In recent years, a number of operations have been devised to treat patients with strokes due to clogging of small arteries. Synthetic tubes are used to connect arteries from the scalp or face to small arteries on the surface of the brain. The benefit of this microvascular surgery is still uncertain.

HEMORRHAGE IN THE BRAIN

Unfortunately, severe high blood pressure can affect the brain in another, much more disastrous way. The increased pressure on their walls causes little arteries and arterioles to burst. Blood then pours into an area of the brain. In addition to developing paralysis, a massive brain hemorrhage can usually lead to coma and often death. Sometimes surgery to remove this blood is indicated, and a neurologist or neurosurgeon should see the patient.

TREATING HIGH BLOOD PRESSURE

We do not know how to prevent high blood pressure, but we certainly know how to treat it. There is almost no one who can't be successfully treated.

Most of the time, we cannot find the exact cause of high blood pressure. We call this condition *essential hypertension*. In a few cases, however, we can find a definite cause and correct it permanently so that the individual does not have to continue taking medication. About 10 percent of the American population has hypertension, and it is obviously not feasible to screen all these people for a few uncommon conditions. Your physician, after he makes a diagnosis of high blood pressure, must determine what tests you need. In all cases, he will want an electrocardiogram and a blood urea test to see whether the high blood pressure has affected your heart or kidneys.

The necessity for other tests depends on your condition. If you are under fifty and have had high blood pressure for only a short time, it may be advisable to check your kidneys more carefully. Sometimes, a clogged artery to the kidney is the cause of high blood pressure. If this artery can be surgically repaired, the high blood pressure may disappear. An intravenous pyelogram (IVP), the same X-ray test that we describe in the chapter on urinary problems (see page 176), can often provide a clue to this diagnosis. If the IVP suggests the presence of a blocked artery, more complicated tests, including an arteriogram, may be appropriate. In the latter test, a dye is injected into an artery in the leg, and X-rays are taken as the dye travels through the kidneys' arteries.

Another even rarer cause of high blood pressure is a benign tumor of the adrenal gland called *pheochromacytoma*. Normally, this gland, which sits right on top of the kidney, makes adrenaline and increases the amount of this hormone in response to exercise or other stress. It enables you to work harder and move faster when you have to. If a tumor develops in the adrenal gland, too much adrenaline comes into the bloodstream and the blood pressure shoots up. Your doctor may suspect this disorder if your blood pressure jumps up and down and if you are a thin, hyperactive person. The tumor can be detected with a urine test that measures breakdown products of adrenaline.

DRUG TREATMENT

Too many people who have high blood pressure are not adequately treated. Successful treatment requires teamwork between doctor and patient. As a patient, you must realize that you will have high blood pressure the rest of your life and you will require lifelong treatment and supervision. The object of treatment is to keep your blood pressure normal without producing serious side effects. You must continue to take your pills conscientiously and regularly even though you feel fine. You are doing this to prevent the kinds of complications we have already discussed. In most cases, once the blood pressure is stabilized, you will probably have to see your physician only about four times a year.

The mainstay of treatment is a water pill (diuretic). This pill eliminates a slight excess of body fluids that may be raising your blood pressure. Before water pills were available, low-salt diets were used in order to keep down the volume of body fluid. However, salt restriction is not effective unless the reduction of salt is so great that food is not palatable. Very few people can stick to such a diet, and so low-salt diets have little to offer in the modern treatment of high blood pressure. In many cases of mild high blood pressure, a water pill taken once or twice a day is sufficient therapy.

Usually it is necessary to add at least one other medication to the water pills. Most of the other medications such as Aldomet (alpha methyl dora), clonidine, and Apresoline (hydralazine) cause the small arterioles to open up (vasodilatation) to let the blood flow more easily and under lower pressure. One drug deserves special mention here because it appears to be very effective. It is called propranolol (Inderal). Propranolol not only causes vasodilatation but also makes the heart beat more quietly and more slowly. Because of its effect on the heart, it is helpful in preventing angina attacks in people who have hardening of the arteries to the heart itself. A combination of propranolol and a water pill will control most cases of high blood pressure.

Propranolol is a very safe drug. It can, however, cause two kinds of trouble. If you already have severe heart trouble, quieting the heartbeat further may aggravate your condition and lead to severe shortness of breath. So your doctor must make sure that your heart is in reasonably good shape before using this drug. People with bronchial asthma may also have trouble if they take propranolol. But for the majority of people with high blood pressure, this drug is an excellent choice.

One word of caution! If you have angina and are taking propranolol, never stop it abruptly. If your doctor feels that you should discontinue using it, he should gradually decrease the dosage over a few days. A few people have had heart attacks when they stopped taking propranolol abruptly.

SIDE EFFECTS OF TREATMENT

One major side effect of high blood pressure treatment is the tendency of the blood pressure to fall too much when you stand up. This leads to dizziness. Each time your doctor examines you, he should check your pressure in the standing as well as lying or sitting positions. If you get dizzy when you stand up, your doctor will make the necessary adjustments in your treatment.

Another serious side effect of blood pressure pills in men is impotence. Many of these drugs may make it difficult or impossible for a man to have an erection. It doesn't happen too often; but when it does, the patient is often too embarrassed to tell his doctor and the doctor frequently forgets to ask or warn the patient in advance. If you do become impotent, tell your doctor immediately. He can always find another drug that will control your blood pressure and relieve you of this unhappy symptom.

SUMMARY

High blood pressure is an extremely common, easily treatable disorder. Since it has potentially devastating consequences, all of us should have our blood pressure checked at least once a year.

7

THE UPS AND DOWNS OF SUGAR IN YOUR BLOOD

If your doctor tells you "You have diabetes," don't panic. Yes, you're going to have to live with it for the rest of your life. But, and it's a very important but, following your doctor's advice, you will be able to live a fairly normal life as millions of diabetics like you are doing every day of their lives all over the world. Naturally, you'll have to run your life somewhat differently from the way your nondiabetic friends run theirs, but, as your doctor will show you, not as differently as you might think.

Diabetes brings some serious complications with it, but most diabetics have none at all or none of the very serious ones.

WHAT IS DIABETES?

Diabetes mellitus has been recognized by physicians for centuries. Literally, it means the "honey urine disease." For a long time, doctors diagnosed diabetes by actually *tasting* their patient's urine. Doctors today do things differently, of course. But essentially the new laboratory tests do what the doctors of old were doing, detecting the presence and amount of sugar in the urine and blood. People with diabetes have a higher than normal level of sugar in their blood, and if it is high enough, sugar spills over into their urine.

This happens because the individual's body is not making enough of a hormone called *insulin*. Insulin is made in the pancreas, an organ in the upper abdomen, and is poured into the bloodstream as the level of sugar in the blood goes up after eating. It lowers the blood sugar primarily by helping the cells to lap up the sugar from the blood and use it for energy.

Insulin has other functions, too. It helps the liver to convert any excessive sugar in the blood into fat and protein for reserve energy and for rebuilding damaged cells. If insulin is not present in the blood in sufficient quantity, the blood sugar concentration keeps rising until it is so high that sugar appears in large quantities in the urine. The body just cannot use this sugar properly as an energy source, and so it passes out of the body in the urine—with very serious consequences. As a result, the individual becomes dehydrated and weak because body cells cannot use the sugar as an energy source. The liver then uses the products of fat breakdown for emergency energy. This results in the formation of certain acids called *ketone bodies*. These ketone bodies make the blood more acid. Body cells cannot function in this acid environment, and so the person becomes sicker and sicker. Left untreated, diabetes can be fatal.

Until the early decades of this century, this was the dismal outlook for many diabetics—rapid loss of strength and death. Then, in 1921 a Canadian scientist, F. G. Banting, and a medical student, Charles Best, isolated insulin from animal pancreases. The discovery and use of insulin proved to be the world's first effective means of treating diabetes. For his work, Banting was knighted by the British government and received the Nobel Prize. Insulin has saved the lives of literally millions of people. The diabetic patient with no insulin of his own can now be managed with proper diet and with insulin injections that he can give himself. He can usually look forward to a normal life.

Fortunately, most diabetic people produce some insulin of their own although not enough to keep their blood-sugar level perfectly normal. In fact, in most people, diabetes is so mild that it causes no symptoms. A doctor will discover diabetes only if he obtains a blood specimen after a meal. A urine test for sugar in mild diabetes may be negative because the sugar level in the blood is not high enough to spill over into the urine. Measurement of blood-sugar levels two hours after a high-carbohydrate meal is the standard screening test for diabetes because we know how high the blood sugar level should be at that time.

Many government and public health organizations run screening drives to detect new diabetics. In fact, each November, the week of Thanksgiving is designated in the United States as "Diabetes Week." Some question the wisdom of this screening. Is it worth the expenditure of large sums of money to detect a disease that will not cause any problems in the majority of the people? This question has caused much controversy. The answer is *yes* only if complications of diabetes can be prevented once the diabetes is detected. As we shall see, some complications may be preventable, but many are not. At any rate, most undetected diabetics will never have any problems.

DIAGNOSIS AND TREATMENT OF DIABETES

If you have very little insulin, you will have warning symptoms of diabetes. You will notice that you must urinate much more frequently and that you are constantly hungry and thirsty. These signs should not be ignored. See your doctor immediately. However, more often than not, diabetes is discovered accidentally in a middle-aged person having blood tests for another reason.

The first rule in the treatment of diabetes is to come down as close as possible to your ideal weight. In fact, if you are overweight, your blood sugar will begin to fall as soon as you start eating less even before you see an appreciable change on the scale. The insulin in your body becomes more effective when confronted with fewer calories.

The next rule has to do with what you eat. The standard diets for diabetes always emphasize cutting down on sugars. Starch, on the other hand, is an acceptable kind of carbohydrate. This means less cake, cookies, and ice cream, but bread, spaghetti, and pasta are okay. The less sugar you consume, the less need there is for insulin.

Detailed diabetic diets telling you what you can eat and how much you can eat are available from several sources, including the American Diabetes Association. The standard diets provide descriptions of model meals and lists of foods that can be substituted for each other. But don't try to use these diets yourself. Your doctor will often use these standard diets, but will modify them to suit your particular needs. He must, for example, take into consideration what it takes to control your blood sugar, the amount of exercise you take, your weight, and other aspects of your life.

With weight loss and reasonable adherence to a diet, most older diabetics need no further therapy for their blood sugar. If your blood sugar is still too high, your doctor can prescribe one of several kinds of pills that will lower your blood sugar further. These pills act by stimulating your pancreas to produce more insulin. They generally do not work in the young diabetic who is incapable of making any insulin. But they are effective in the majority of people who become diabetic after the age of fifty.

Finally, if your blood sugar remains very high despite the above measures, your doctor will prescribe insulin injections. After a little instruction, you will easily be able to give yourself these daily injections. Most of the time, the doctor will prescribe a long-acting insulin such as NPH or Lente insulin, which you will take only once daily, in the morning.

HOW MUCH CONTROL OF BLOOD SUGAR?

At this point, we must deal with an important controversy that surrounds the treatment of diabetes. Many people think that all the answers in medicine are clear cut. Actually, in many areas our knowledge is still inadequate, and doctors, naturally, disagree with each other. There is no subject in medicine that arouses more spirited arguments than the treatment of diabetes. First, we aren't sure what is a low enough and safe enough blood sugar level for the diabetic. We know it is very difficult to keep the diabetic's blood sugar count perfectly normal all the time. If we try to do this, his blood sugar may drop too far and lead to brain damage. We do not know whether it is really important to our health to have a blood sugar very close to normal. Many doctors feel that it is necessary only to keep it from reaching a dangerously high level.

Second, there are some serious objections to the use of pills that lower blood sugar. A study compared how well diabetics did with and without these pills and came to the conclusion that those who took these pills had more fatal heart attacks. However, many experts have challenged the methods in this study that they feel make the results invalid. So a doctor treating a patient with diabetes is often faced with a dilemma. If the patient's blood sugar is still moderately high after he has lost weight and has followed a diet, should he prescribe the pills, should he have the patient inject himself with insulin every day, or should he leave the blood sugar alone? Any two competent, thoughtful doctors could give quite different answers to these questions.

In medicine it is always important to do no harm where you can do no good. Those doctors who try to keep the blood-sugar level very close to normal are hoping that this will prevent the complications of diabetes. So far, however, there is very little evidence to support this hope, particularly in older people. The authors prefer the cautious treatment. We prefer to use diabetic pills sparingly and settle for moderate control of the blood sugar through weight loss and diet. Of course, if patients don't follow our dietary suggestions, we have no choice. We must prescribe insulin or pills. If the blood sugar remains high and ketone bodies appear in the urine, you must receive insulin.

Experts still cannot agree on a definition of diabetes in older people. We have tended to define a diabetic as a person with blood-sugar levels higher than normal. The "normal" blood-sugar level was established by doing blood-sugar level tests on young people in their twenties. We know, however, that it is normal for blood-sugar levels to rise with age, and so people in their sixties and seventies may have rather high levels without really being diabetic. Furthermore, certain drugs such as water pills (diuretics) raise the blood sugar, and these pills are often prescribed for older people. This difficulty in determining diabetes in older people is really another reason for following cautious, conservative treatment. We feel it makes no sense to prescribe potent medicines or even radical changes in diet for a person in his sixties or seventies whose blood-sugar level is only moderately high.

LIVING WITH DIABETES

If you do require treatment for diabetes, you cannot just take your medication and forget about it. You have a lifelong disorder requiring lifelong preventive measures. You can, however, certainly lead a perfectly normal life, provided you are checked by your doctor periodically and you follow his advice and treatment faithfully. You and he are partners for life.

You must know that your blood-sugar level may be affected by many things, by your psychological state, for example. Anxiety or emotional strain may cause your blood-sugar level to go up. Infections of any kind, even a cold, may also increase your body's need for insulin and raise the blood-sugar level. On the other hand, if you have a stomach virus that makes you vomit and stop eating, you may need less insulin. Your usual dose of medicine might lower the blood sugar too much.

For all of these reasons, diabetes severe enough to treat is severe enough to be watched closely. Your doctor will teach you how to inject insulin if you need it. He will also teach you how to check for sugar in your urine. This can be done simply by one of several commercial methods. The easiest involves dipping a specially treated strip of paper into the urine and watching for a color change that occurs within seconds. The color is compared with a color chart to determine how much sugar is present. If you do this twice daily, you and your doctor will have a pretty good idea of how your blood sugar is running. A sudden change may be a warning that something is wrong and that you should see your doctor sooner.

No matter what the urine test shows, you should always check with your doctor if you do not feel right for a few days. Increasing thirst, frequent urination, or stomach symptoms may indicate that you are becoming dehydrated because your blood sugar is too high. If you are vomiting or not eating, check with your doctor about your dose of medicine. Feelings of weakness, faintness, or restlessness may be signs of too low a blood sugar. Episodes of sudden sweating and dizziness must always be taken seriously. Call your doctor at once.

COMPLICATIONS

There are two kinds of complications in diabetes: 1) those that are peculiar to diabetes and 2) those that occur more commonly in diabetics than nondiabetics. We must emphasize at the outset that most people with diabetes do not develop any complications. If you are diabetic, you can look forward to leading a perfectly normal life. Even some of the finest professional athletes have been diabetic. Nevertheless, a diabetic person should know something about what can happen because of his disease and what can be done to prevent complications.

The most specific complication of diabetes is a weakening of the lining of the very smallest blood vessels—arterioles and capillaries. These little vessels become porous and leak either blood or fluid from the bloodstream into the surrounding area. The leaky capillary is the hallmark of diabetes and can be seen under the microscope in the skin of some diabetic people even before their blood-sugar levels get too high. Fortunately, these microscopic changes rarely become widespread or severe enough to cause any problems. When they do, signs and symptoms may occur in a number of places. The most common problems arise in the eyes and kidneys.

EYE PROBLEMS

Diabetes is now the leading cause of blindness in the United States. Its major target in the eye is the retina (see chapter 18). The retina is made up of very sensitive cells that record light images and transmit them to the brain via the optic nerve. The retina is very easily damaged by any abnormal stress. When the capillaries that deliver blood to the retina become porous (microaneurysm) fluid and blood leak out, stretching and swelling the retina. If this occurs frequently enough, there may be irreversible damage, and parts of the retina wear out. In addition, these porous capillaries do not deliver sufficient oxygen to the retina. Lack of oxygen leads to scars that may destroy the retina (*retinitis proliferans*).

Most diabetics who have some bleeding in their retinas will not become blind, but they are certainly at greater risk. Your doctor can spot obvious changes in your retina when he routinely examines your eyes, but very early changes can be found only with sophisticated tests performed by an eye specialist (ophthalmologist).

What can be done to prevent blindness from retinal damage? Until recently, very little. But now we are in a much better position to do something positive. First of all, we know that diabetics with normal blood pressures have much less trouble with their eyes than those with elevated pressures. We also know that high blood pressure occurs very frequently in diabetic people. So it's very important that every diabetic have his blood pressure checked several times a year. If it is up, prompt treatment plays an important part in preventing eye trouble.

Secondly, we have a new technique for treating retinal damage. We have learned how to use laser beams to help the damaged eye. Eye doctors specializing in this therapy can direct a very narrow beam to almost any spot on the retina. This beam can burn out damaged blood vessels and porous capillaries and prevent retinal damage. This technique is amazingly precise and can be performed without damaging normal parts of the retina. Of course, it is obviously a major decision that is taken only for people with serious retinal damage and only after careful consultation with the appropriate specialists.

If you are diabetic, have your eyes checked regularly by an ophthalmologist. We suggest a visit every six months if you have no retinal damage, and even more often if you are having retinal problems.

The ophthalmologist has special instruments for looking at your retina and can pick up early, reversible changes. If he is not sure of what he is seeing, he may ask for a special test called *fluorescein angiography*. In this test, a green dye is injected into a vein, and a movie is taken of the retina as the dye goes through the arteries and capillaries. The movie will show abnormalities in capillaries and leakage that is not visible by any other method.

In addition to retinal damage, diabetes can lead to loss of vision through formation of cataracts (see chapter 18). The frequency of cataracts is much higher in diabetics than in nondiabetics. Fortunately, surgical removal of these cataracts is easy, and results are excellent. If your vision is decreasing or becoming blurry, cataracts are the first things your doctor will look for.

KIDNEY TROUBLE

The capillaries and small blood vessels of the kidneys may be involved in the same way that the eyes are involved. This causes the blood and blood proteins to pass through into the urine in the early stage and can lead to kidney failure in the more advanced stages. Unfortunately, we have no definite way of preventing this kidney problem. Some authorities believe that control of blood sugar will decrease the likelihood of kidney damage, but there is no solid proof for this theory. Treatment for diabetic kidney damage is similar to treatment of other kidney diseases: proper diet, good fluid intake, and in the late stages, use of the artificial kidney (chronic hemodialysis, see page 177).

NERVE PROBLEMS

Perhaps the most common of the specific complications of diabetes is damage to nerves (*neuritis*). In fact, almost all diabetics eventually have some damage to the ends of some nerves although this damage is usually not severe enough to cause any symptoms. This form of neuritis rarely affects the nerves to muscles, and so your muscle strength remains normal. It is the nerves that carry sensation that are damaged, the nerves in the feet being the most affected. Some diabetics complain of intermittent "pins and needles" sensation in their toes and fingers or that their feet fall asleep. Occasionally, they have shooting pains in their legs. These pains subside with time.

In the more severe cases, neuritis can lead to gradual loss of sensation. If this loss is very severe, your feet may become quite numb. In fact, you may not be able to feel heat, cold, pain, or even a light touch. Thus, your doctor's periodic examination should include carefully checking sensation in your feet.

If your feet do not respond properly to heat, cold, or pain, you can easily injure them without knowing it. Bath water, for example, may feel very comfortable to you when it is really burning your feet. For this reason, we instruct all diabetic people to look at their feet regularly and even use a mirror to inspect the soles, to check bath and shower water with their elbows, and never to use hot-water bottles or electric blankets on their feet.

After sensation has been absent for a long time, painless open ulcers may develop on the soles of the feet. They are caused by excessive pressure, which is ordinarily prevented by reflex movement of your feet. If you lose sensation, you lose these reflexes and put too much weight on one area of the foot for prolonged periods. You can recognize a trouble spot early by the formation of thickened skin on the sole just behind the toes. This thick skin (callus) should be treated regularly by a podiatrist. The podiatrist can also prescribe a special shoe that will take the pressure off the area of callus. Be sure that the podiatrist knows that you have diabetes before he begins to treat you. As we pointed out earlier, diabetics often have decreased circulation in their feet. The podiatrist must take this into account in working on your feet. Of course, all the foot-care instructions that we mentioned earlier in the chapter on circulation (see page 5) apply to every diabetic person.

Occasionally, the neuritis can involve the nerves that go to internal organs. The reflex that keeps your blood pressure from falling when you stand up may not work properly. If you stand up too quickly, you may feel lightheaded or dizzy because your brain temporarily is not receiving enough blood. This is generally not serious and can be avoided by getting up more slowly. If you have more severe dizziness, your doctor can prescribe elastic stockings that will force blood from your legs to your brain.

Other possible effects of the nerve damage include difficulty in urinating, occasional diarrhea, and, in men, impotence.

It is very important for diabetics to take particularly good care of their feet. Here is what the diabetic must do to protect his feet from injury:

1. Check bath or shower water with your elbows to make sure that it is lukewarm.
2. Look at your feet at least twice a week to make sure that there are no breaks in the skin. Use a mirror to inspect your soles.
3. Do not use heating pads or electric blankets on your feet.
4. Wear comfortable, well-fitted shoes. Made-to-order, orthopedic shoes are not necessary unless you are developing pressure sores or ulcers on your feet.
5. Have regular care by a podiatrist who knows that you are diabetic. The podiatrist, rather than you, should cut your toenails when necessary. The podiatrist should also care for any calluses or pressure areas and recommend special shoes when necessary to relieve undue pressure.
6. Do not smoke.

SWELLING

A less common complication of diabetes is the development of swelling of the legs and other parts of the body (*edema*). This happens because fluid from the bloodstream leaks through damaged capillaries into the body's tissues. After a few days, this fluid is taken back into the bloodstream and the swelling disappears. These changes are paralleled by weight changes. Swelling causes weight gain. When the fluid goes back into the bloodstream and is eliminated by the kidneys, the weight goes down again. Sometimes, the swelling is distributed so evenly throughout the body that you may notice only the change in weight. Unexplained fluctuations in weight, therefore, may be the first sign of diabetes.

ARTERIOSCLEROSIS

By far the most serious threat to the diabetic is arteriosclerosis (hardening of the arteries, see Chapter 1), which may develop at a relatively early age. This arteriosclerosis makes the diabetic more vulnerable than the nondiabetic to heart attacks, strokes, and circulatory problems in the legs. Unfortunately, control of the blood-sugar level has no apparent effect on arteriosclerosis and the problems it brings with it.

What can you do to prevent arteriosclerosis? You cannot get rid of your diabetes, but you can try to decrease or eliminate other risk factors. We have discussed these before, but they are worth repeating briefly here:

1. Keep your weight down as close as possible to what your weight was at full maturity (about age twenty-five).
2. Try to avoid saturated fats such as in cake, ice cream, organ meats, and red meats.
3. Have your blood pressure checked regularly.
4. Do not smoke.
5. Lead an active life with regular, moderate exercise.

LOW BLOOD SUGAR

Many laymen are under the false impression that low blood sugar (*hypoglycemia*) is a common problem. Not so. Significant hypoglycemia is not at all frequent except in people with diabetes who take too much insulin or too many blood-sugar-lowering pills.

Low blood-sugar levels, when they do occur, can cause a variety of symptoms that differ from person to person. These symptoms fall into two main categories. The most important effects are felt by the brain, which cannot function without a continuous supply of sugar. Unlike other areas of the body, brain cells cannot break down fat or protein for use as fuel; they can use only sugar. Therefore, a person with a low blood-sugar level may experience mental confusion, dizziness, weakness, tiredness, fainting, and coma. Low blood sugar may also lead to emotional changes such as anger, depression, and strange behavior. Blood-sugar levels are among the first laboratory tests that your doctor will order if you have any of these symptoms. In fact, any one found unconscious should immediately receive an intravenous injection of sugar (glucose) solution just in case he has a low blood-sugar level.

The other symptoms of hypoglycemia are related to the body's attempt to bring the sugar level back up to normal. Certain chemical messengers (hormones) have, as one of their jobs, raising the blood-sugar level, and protecting against too much insulin. One of the most powerful and quick-acting hormones in this regard is adrenaline. As soon as the blood sugar falls below normal, adrenaline is poured into the bloodstream and causes sugar stored in the liver to come into the bloodstream. Adrenaline also has other effects, such as closing small blood vessels in the skin and increasing sweating. Many people having a hypoglycemic attack, therefore, feel cold and clammy and sweat profusely. A cold sweat then is often a clue to a hypoglycemic attack.

CAUSES OF LOW BLOOD SUGAR

The treatment of hypoglycemia depends on its cause. If overtreatment of diabetes is the cause, the doctor will cut back on the medication. If you are not diabetic and you have symptoms that can be due to hypoglycemia, your doctor will look for several possible causes. The serious causes all tend to produce hypoglycemia when you have not eaten for a number of hours. This fasting hypoglycemia may be caused by thyroid gland or adrenal gland deficiency, liver problems, alcoholism, or a tumor of the pancreas that produces too much insulin. Your doctor must perform special tests to find the exact cause and treat you accordingly.

On the other hand, the most common kind of hypoglycemia occurs a few hours after eating and is generally very easy to handle. In this situation, an overactive pancreas makes too much insulin in response to a carbohydrate meal. If you have this problem, you can prevent low blood-sugar attacks by eating smaller meals and restricting your intake of carbohydrates.

The following table summarizes the causes and treatment of low blood sugar:

CAUSE	TREATMENT
1. Overtreatment for diabetes: taking too much insulin, etc.	1. Cut back on medication.
2. Overactive pancreas responds to a carbohydrate meal with too much insulin.	2. Eat smaller meals and cut down on carbohydrates.
3. People with liver disease or alcoholics who have not eaten for twenty-four hours: their liver cannot supply emergency rations of sugar to the bloodstream. Normal people can fast for seventy-two	3. Avoid alcohol and eat regularly.

hours without exhibiting
signs of hypoglycemia.

4. Deficiency of the thyroid
or adrenal glands that
deprives the body of hor-
mones that raise blood-
sugar levels.

4. Thyroid or cortisone pills.

5. Tumor of pancreas
(rare).

5. Surgical removal of the
tumor.

SUMMARY

1. Diabetes is one of the oldest diseases known to man.

2. Diabetes is extremely common. Three to 5 percent of
the American population has diabetes although millions are
not aware of it.

3. The basic problem in diabetes is a deficiency of a
hormone called insulin. When the pancreas does not produce enough insulin, the level of sugar in the bloodstream
rises.

4. Increasing need to urinate and drink fluids may be
the first symptom of diabetes. More often, diabetes is discovered accidentally when blood tests are performed for
other reasons.

5. Although there is no cure at this time, diabetes can
be controlled with diet, pills, and insulin injections if necessary.

6. Diabetics develop many complications, such as eye,
kidney, nerve problems, and premature arteriosclerosis. Fortunately, most diabetic people do not suffer from these
problems.

7. Every diabetic should pay particular attention to his
feet and have a thorough eye examination at least twice a
year.

8

WHEN YOUR STOMACH MISBEHAVES

Digestive problems are the one truly common bond of suffering linking all of us of all ages. Neither young nor old can escape them. Many people think our intestines grow more difficult to live with as the years go by, but on the whole they serve us quite well. In fact, in many ways our intestines hold up better than the rest of our organs. This may seem hard to believe considering all the complaints of "poor digestion" from older friends or relatives. But there are many reasons for this, often having nothing at all to do with the intestines: other factors, such as loneliness, boredom, unlimited free time in which to dwell on vague complaints most of us ignore, and at times, a simple need for attention. Least expressed, but very often present, however, is the very real fear of cancer, heightened by the well-publicized "danger signs" of cancer.

We shall now take a closer look at some of the most commonly encountered complaints.

INDIGESTION

Everyone knows what indigestion is, but no one seems to be able to describe it. Most descriptions that one hears are better suited to the medieval torture rack: "burning," "cutting," "bloating," "twisting." The common theme, however, is distress in the upper abdomen, often appearing around mealtime. It is not unusual to experience some digestive discomfort after excessive eating. Yet we seem to recall that when we were younger we were able to devour virtually anything that resembled food without the slightest rebuff from our digestive tract.

Actually, our ability to digest our food does change as we grow older. There are many reasons for this. Certainly changes in food preferences play a role, as does a reduced level of physical activity and poor teeth. Furthermore, mealtime is no longer an important social event. No doubt other factors, such as ill health, multiple drug use, and the simple need for fewer calories, all contribute to changed appetites in older people.

Chronic indigestion shouldn't be ignored at any age. On the contrary, you should discuss these symptoms with your doctor. If they have been present for a long time without much change, he may decide to treat them with simple measures. On the other hand, recent symptoms or symptoms that seem to be increasing in frequency or severity may require further investigation. Frequently this entails an upper GI series, a special X-ray of the intestinal tract taken while drinking a milky liquid called *barium*. This test can usually spot such problems as tumors or ulcers.

Because an X-ray is merely a photograph of the barium-coated intestine, it is really an indirect method of examination—an analysis of shadows. Thus, if your doctor still has doubts, he may suggest a more sophisticated procedure called *gastroscopy* or *upper GI endoscopy*. By means of a flexible tube that you swallow, or that is inserted with a local anesthetic, the specialist who performs this test can look directly into your stomach and upper intestine and see clearly many problems the X-ray misses. With this instru-

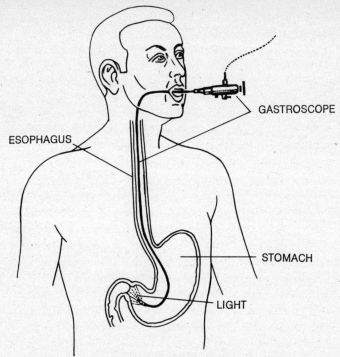

Fig. 18   Illustration of gastroscopy. The esophagus, stomach, and duodenum can all be seen by this procedure. This is why it is also
called esophogogastroduodenoscopy.

ment, it is also possible to take small pieces of tissue from
any unhealthy appearing area to be examined later under
the microscope. It is even possible now to remove small
polyps or growths through this instrument.

OTHER TESTS FOR INDIGESTION

There are other tests that your doctor can call upon if he
is not satisfied that he has gotten to the root of the problem.
For example, he may wish to order some tests to check for
gall bladder problems (see page 132). These are simple
tests.

The situation is more complicated if he suspects that
your indigestion is caused by a problem in your pancreas.
This is an elongated organ buried deep in the abdomen and

snuggled tightly against the spine. It produces both important digestive juices and the hormone *insulin*. Because of its inaccessibility, the pancreas is one of the most difficult organs to examine. It can become inflamed in people with gall bladder problems, and injury to the pancreas often occurs in people who drink large quantities of alcohol over a long period.

Sudden injury to the pancreas is called *pancreatitis*. This usually begins with severe abdominal pain that often travels straight through to the back. A simple blood test (*serum amylase*) usually confirms the diagnosis.

Tumors of the pancreas, however, are much harder to diagnose. Fortunately, newer techniques now permit more thorough, virtually painless examination of the pancreas than was ever possible before. One of these methods called *ultrasound* is able to form images of the gall bladder and pancreas by means of high-frequency sound waves. Another specialized form of X-ray, the whole body scanner (*CAT scan*) is able to reconstruct an image of the abdominal or-

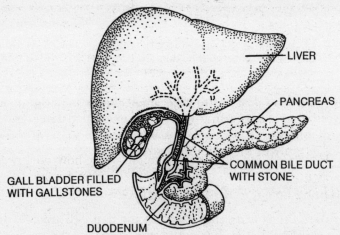

Fig. 19   Normal relationship of liver, gall bladder, bile ducts, pancreas, and intestine (duodenum). Bile made in the liver and stored in the gall bladder flows through the common bile duct into the duodenum. Note that the duct from the pancreas joins the common bile duct just before entering the duodenum. In this illustration, gallstones are shown in the gall bladder where they are blocking the bile duct. With bile trapped behind the stone, jaundice would probably be present.

gans using a computer and provides reliable information about the appearance of the pancreas. Ultrasound tests are now widely available in most hospitals, but the prohibitive cost of the computerized whole-body scanner limits its use to a few specialized centers.

The pancreas can also be visualized by injections of dye into its arteries, but this is a more cumbersome and uncomfortable technique. Sometimes it is helpful to measure the quantity of the digestive juices that the pancreas produces using a small rubber tube that is swallowed or inserted with a local anesthetic. The juice can also be examined for abnormal cells. Another technique that can be used for examining the pancreas is called by the imposing name of *endoscopic retrograde cholongio-pancreatography* (or "ERCP" for short, see page 136). It is important to realize that no diagnostic procedure is completely accurate. So it may be necessary to undergo several.

We have discussed these tests at great length to illustrate the difficulties your doctor encounters when he suspects a serious problem and looks for the cause. And these do not even take into account many of the other possible reasons for abdominal discomfort that he confronts daily.

Fortunately, however, it is rarely necessary to go to such great lengths in seeking a reason for indigestion. In most cases, a few simple tests will do. Moreover, even after thorough examination, it is not unusual for the doctor to be left without knowing the precise cause. This does not reflect on your doctor's competence, nor should it lead you to doubt that your complaints are real.

We simply do not know enough about how our intestines behave to come up with an explanation for all symptoms in the absence of some visible abnormality. This is very often the case when the complaint is indigestion.

What makes your doctor decide to embark on a thorough examination or to first try a simple treatment? Generally, if the symptoms are merely annoying and have fluctuated over the years without much change, it is reasonable to postpone a prolonged and often tiresome and uncomfortable investigation. On the other hand, new pain, or acceleration of symptoms, weight loss, or any unexplainable finding on physical examination or lab test may be enough to cause your doctor to look further.

One symptom that seems to go hand in hand with indigestion is bloating or belching. This is rarely a sign of a serious problem. It is usually caused by excessive air swallowing either as a nervous habit or as an intentional maneuver to relieve a sense of fullness. Eating and especially drinking too quickly, drinking carbonated beverages, chewing gum, or nervous swallowing of saliva usually account for most cases of belching. Once the causes are recognized, it is usually possible to correct the habits that lead to this complaint.

LIVING WITH INDIGESTION

Most people with indigestion will find that there is nothing seriously wrong with them. Somewhat surprisingly, they often receive this news with more disappointment than relief. They cannot believe that all their symptoms are not only harmless but are not even caused by a physically describable condition. To meet this problem, the doctor may refer to some minor abnormality he found during the examination, or resort to an all-embracing term like "gastritis." Not that such a condition does not exist. Gastritis, which, simply put, is an inflammation of the lining of the stomach, is a very common condition, often noticed incidentally by specialists who look into the stomach. But this almost invariably develops as we grow older and rarely causes symptoms. Nevertheless, it is reassuring to know that your orphaned symptoms have found themselves a place of refuge in the medical lexicon.

The more important problem is how to best deal with the digestive complaints once you have been cleared by your doctor. Here are a few suggestions.

1. Reconcile yourself to the fact you are going to have some occasional stomach upsets. This does not mean that something is seriously wrong with you. When you go into any supermarket these days, you can't help noticing those long aisles filled with medicines for indigestion and heart-

burn. This is an indication of how common this problem really is. Yet most people learn to live with their minor stomach upsets, and so can you.

2. Stick to regular eating habits. When you are no longer held to a rigid time schedule, you'll develop a tendency to skip meals. To make matters worse, you may even neglect the main meal, which no longer includes the anticipation of a lively family gathering. While it is easy to understand that a good meal is not as enjoyable without the company of friends and family, it is important to realize that the meal itself is essential. So try to stick with regular meal hours, which should include at least one full, well-balanced meal.

3. Eat slowly and chew your food well. Much of the gassy feeling after eating comes from swallowing too much air with your meal as you eat hurriedly. Take your time. You'll improve your digestion and enjoy your meal more.

4. Try to pinpoint the foods that give you trouble. You know which foods disagree with you. As we grow older, certain kinds of foods commonly lead to discomfort: fried and fatty foods, raw fruits and vegetables, coffee. The commonly held notion that certain foods such as the legumes (beans) can cause gas, is in fact, correct. So if you're bloated and gassy, switch to broiled lean meats and well-cooked vegetables.

5. Eat a well-balanced diet (see page 169). This means meat and vegetables and dairy products. If nothing especially appeals to you, try some variety in cooking. You may discover as much enjoyment in the preparing as in the eating.

6. Don't be discouraged if you don't have the same craving for food that you once had. This is normal. Actually, with regular eating habits, you may recapture your delight in a good meal.

7. What about all those chalky, sweet liquids people take for indigestion? Do they help? It is doubtful that they really do more than eliminate some acid. Some people find that a tablespoon of the liquid has a soothing effect. If it works for you, fine. Don't use them regularly without con-

sulting your doctor. In small doses, they are perfectly safe, but large quantities over an extended period of time can lead to problems.

8. What we have been discussing about indigestion up to now assumes that you have been checked by your doctor to be certain that you have no serious problems. Don't be ashamed about seeking help just because friends or relatives have similar complaints or make light of your distress. They may be right, but only your doctor can say for sure. See your doctor right away if you have any of the following symptoms.

a) Discomfort which is persistent or increases in severity or frequency
b) Weight loss
c) Change in bowel habits
d) Difficulty in swallowing
e) Vomiting
f) Jaundice (yellowing of the eyes or skin).

HEARTBURN

In most peoples' minds heartburn and indigestion are so closely linked that the terms are used interchangeably to identify a type of distress that everyone has experienced. After all, our gastrointestinal tract has only a limited number of symptoms to call for help when something is amiss. Unfortunately, the discomfort it uses to alert you to its distress may be the same for minor and major conditions.

We have already defined indigestion as any sense of discomfort or pain in the abdomen, generally related to meals. While the symptom itself will be of little help to your doctor in making an immediate diagnosis, it does provide the common ground for both of you to begin to work on your problem.

For this reason it is useful to look upon "heartburn" as a symptom distinct from indigestion. Heartburn usually indicates a specific problem if we stick to a strict definition of a "burning" sensation beginning in the lower part of the chest beneath the breastbone and traveling upward toward the neck. This can be associated with an acid taste in the mouth and made worse by lying down or bending. This burning sensation is caused by the backflow of stomach acid into the *esophagus* or swallowing tube. Normally, stomach juices are prevented from splashing backward into the esophagus by a valvelike barrier at the lower end of the esophagus. When this barrier fails, acid floods the sensitive lining of the esophagus producing the sensation long referred to as "heartburn." Just about everyone has experienced this sensation at one time or another. The valve is not effective at all times but the small amount of acid that may leak backward on occasion is usually swept immediately into the stomach. The discomfort is usually temporary. Most of the time it is our fault for overeating or eating food we know will offend our digestive tract.

If the condition occurs regularly, and particularly when lying down or even stooping, chances are that the valve, or *sphincter*, as it is called, is not functioning effectively and is allowing acid from the stomach to bathe the sensitive esophageal lining. A *hiatus hernia* often accompanies this *acid reflux*, as it is called, although not always. A hiatus hernia

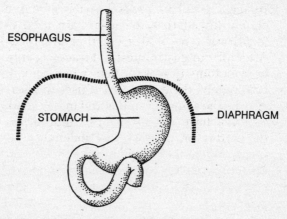

Fig. 20 Normal relationship of esophagus and stomach to the diaphragm. Note that the stomach and a small portion of esophagus lie below the diaphragm.

is one of the most common problems doctors discover on upper GI series (see page 116). Fortunately, in the majority of cases, it is an innocent condition, probably related to some weakening of tissues with age, although there are certainly younger people with this condition.

Just what is a hiatus hernia? It is easy to understand if you remember that our chest, which contains the lungs and heart, is separated from the abdomen by a dividing shelf called the *diaphragm* (see Fig 20). The esophagus, or swallowing tube, in the chest reaches the stomach through an opening in the diaphragm. Ordinarily, the stomach remains anchored in the abdomen below the diaphragm. If it should slip loose from its moorings, it will ascend partly into the chest through this hole in the diaphragm. Actually this rarely causes problems and most people will never know that they have a hiatus hernia. Does the hernia itself cause any trouble? Not very often and then usually when most of the stomach slips into the chest, but even here it may not cause symptoms.

Since, with time, the stomach acid can have a corrosive

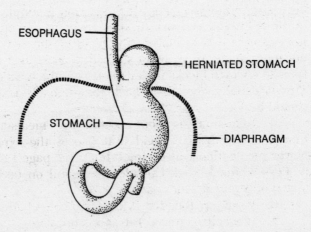

Fig. 21   Hiatus hernia. Note that a portion of the stomach now lies above the diaphragm.

effect on the delicate esophageal lining, a few people may develop more serious consequences such as bleeding or narrowing of the esophagus, which can hamper swallowing. For most people, however, heartburn is the chief problem they will have to deal with. If you follow a few simple rules, you should be able to control the symptoms of heartburn.

1. Anything that increases pressure in the abdomen will make the heartburn worse. So avoid eating rapidly. Chew carefully, and don't eat too much at one sitting.

2. Too much air in the stomach worsens the heartburn. So make a conscious effort to stop swallowing air. For the same reason, keep away from carbonated beverages, chewing gum, and hard candies.

3. Tight belts, girdles, or pants may halt that outward advance of your belly but they put increasing pressure on your stomach. So if your symptoms are giving you trouble, try a loose belt and discard that girdle.

4. When you're lying down, stomach juices will flow with gravity toward the esophagus. Ordinarily, the valve acts as a dam to break this flow. When the sphincter is weakened, acid will flow unimpeded into the esophagus. This is the reason that many people experience severe heartburn after going to bed or after bending. A simple maneuver to allow gravity to work in your favor by directing gastric juices forward is to elevate the head of the bed. This does not mean using more pillows. Just raise the bed by putting four- to six-inch blocks under the legs at the head of the bed. This is usually enough to keep the stomach acid where it should be.

5. Take antacids about an hour after meals and at bedtime to neutralize the acid that causes the symptoms. A newer medication called cimetidine (see page 128), which reduces stomach acid, can also be useful on occasion, but take it only on a doctor's advice.

6. Avoid any food for at least two hours before retiring.

7. Avoid citrus juices, fats, and chocolate.

In most people, these simple measures are enough to relieve the heartburn. For those few who seem unable to obtain relief or who develop severe inflammation of the esophagus, surgery may have to be considered. This is not the usual situation, however, and satisfying results are usually achieved with simple treatment.

TROUBLE WITH SWALLOWING

To reach the stomach, food must pass through a small muscular tube called the esophagus (see Fig. 20). When you drink cold water, you can actually feel the liquid descending in your chest and entering your stomach. Food is carried through this tube by a gentle kneading movement. This is why you can actually eat upside down, although we obviously do not recommend this dinner-table posture. If the food meets an obstacle in its slow descent down the esophagus, pressure rises to squeeze it past. This abnormal pressure head can be quite painful as anyone can appreciate who has hurriedly swallowed an oversized piece of food and suffered its agonizing journey down the esophagus.

Normally, as we eat, we give little thought to swallowing and are not aware of the passage of food into our stomachs. If the food should meet some obstacle that hinders its normally smooth passage, you will experience a sense of "sticking" in the chest. If food seems to "stick" every time you eat, especially if it seems to worsen, see your doctor. This sensation is not normal. It can be caused by abnormal squeezing of the esophagus or by an actual mechanical interference to the flow of food as a tumor, or scarring of the esophagus due to inflammation. In the latter case, it may be possible to stretch the narrowed scarred area called a *stricture*. This usually develops in people who have had heartburn with reversed flow of acid for many years.

To find the cause of problems with swallowing, all that may be required is a barium X-ray study. Often endoscopy (see page 116) will clarify the problem. Detection of abnormal squeezing problems may require swallowing small tubes to measure pressure waves in the esophagus. This latter test is not available everywhere. Your doctor will decide just how thorough an examination your particular problem deserves.

PEPTIC ULCER

The first thought that crosses most people's minds when they experience persistent stomach pains and indigestion is "I have an ulcer." Most of the time this turns out not to be the case. An ulcer is a break in the lining of the upper part of the intestines, looking very much like a canker sore in the mouth. The words "peptic ulcer" indicate that the ulcer is located in an area bathed by the acid juices of the stomach. To be specific, the ulcer should be named according to its exact location. Gastric ulcers occur in the stomach, while duodenal ulcers develop in the small portion of the intestine immediately adjacent to the stomach.

The typical pain of ulcer is a burning, gnawing sensation in the pit of the stomach appearing about an hour after meals or on an empty stomach. The ulcer pain is relieved by food. Often the pain awakens a person several hours after retiring. In older people, however, the pain may not be this precise, and, in fact, may lead the doctors astray by its unusual or nondescript quality.

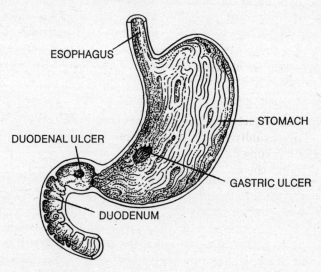

Fig. 22   Illustration of typical location of peptic ulcers. The ulcer in the stomach is called a gastric ulcer.

Gastric ulcers are viewed with greater concern by most physicians than duodenal ulcers. For reasons not understood, gastric ulcers are much more common in older people. One of the reasons that gastric ulcers receive greater attention than duodenal ulcers is the occasional problem of establishing with certainty that the ulcer is completely benign, not cancerous. This problem does not arise with duodenal ulcers, which, for all practical purposes, are never malignant (cancerous). With use of modern techniques, however, especially *fiberoptic endoscopy* (see page 116), the doctor can feel assured that he knows the problem he is dealing with. The barium X-ray examination will provide adequate information in most cases. If there is any doubt about whether an ulcer is present or about its seriousness, a gastroscopic examination should resolve the issue.

Peptic ulcers have earned the ill-deserved reputation of seeking out young, aggressive, anxiety-prone individuals, but the majority of ulcer patients do not fit this category. In fact, ulcers are just as common in older people, and, as we have indicated, gastric ulcers are even more frequent among them.

What causes an ulcer? While we don't have all the answers, it is quite clear that acid produced by the stomach plays an important part. We know that ulcers cannot develop in the absence of acid, and they heal promptly when the acid is neutralized. Yet this is not the whole story since many people without ulcers produce more acid than people with ulcers. Ulcers also seem to run in families.

TREATMENT OF ULCER

Ulcers can thrive only in an acid environment. When the acid is reduced, the ulcer will slowly shrink and heal. The standard treatment for many decades involved neutralizing the acid with liquid buffers (antacids). Since acid is continually made by the stomach, and these buffers are rapidly expelled, it is necessary to take large quantities frequently over a long period of time. Since the food we eat will buffer stomach acids, it has not been necessary to use these antacids at mealtime. Recently a medication in pill form, called *cimetidine*, has been marketed with a great deal of fanfare.

It inhibits the stomach from manufacturing acid and has the distinct advantage of requiring only four doses daily. It is doubtful that it is any more effective than the traditional antacids taken every two hours. Nonetheless, most people prefer the convenience of a tablet taken only a few times a day rather than carrying about unwieldy bottles of antacid that must be taken frequently.

As a rule, doctors keep gastric ulcers under closer scrutiny than duodenal ulcers and many specialists actually prefer to confirm complete healing of a gastric ulcer by repeating the gastroscopy after a month or two. Duodenal ulcers are assumed to heal and are not as intensively observed.

Unfortunately, many ulcers will recur, particularly duodenal ulcers. When they do, they are treated just the same as before.

SURGERY FOR ULCER

There are times when surgery seems to be the most effective way to deal with a problem ulcer. When the disabling pain of ulcer recurs year after year, or when it continues unabated for weeks on end with no relief in sight, the ulcer is said to be intractable to medical management. Up until now this has been the most common reason for resorting to surgery.

While surgery may be chosen subjectively, that is, on the basis of persistent discomfort that one is unable to bear any longer, there are occasions when surgery is the only alternative, as when the ulcer perforates (breaks through) the bowel wall, a critical situation that calls for immediate action. The same goes for an ulcer that continues to bleed for many hours posing a direct threat to life. If an ulcer has bled repeatedly over the years, it also seems wise to consider surgery. Experience has shown that once an ulcer has bled it is likely to bleed again, with probabilities increasing with each succeeding episode. Each bleeding episode carries with it a definite risk.

An ulcer that heals by constant scarring may ultimately block the passage of food from the stomach into the intestines. Here, too, surgery is usually the most satisfactory means of correcting the problem.

Gastric ulcer poses a unique problem, not associated with duodenal ulcers. This is the question of malignancy and constant need for follow-up. So concerned are some doctors that they do not hesitate to advise surgery under circumstances that would not even be considered for duodenal ulcer. Still, with current methods that provide more detailed oversight of gastric ulcers, there seems to be less reluctance to pursue medical treatment. Obviously, just as with duodenal ulcers, when a life-threatening complication arises, surgery may be the only alternative.

Interestingly, with the better patient compliance afforded by the new tablets for treatment of ulcers, there seems to be a decrease in the number of operations being performed for treatment of peptic ulcers in general, and specifically for duodenal ulcer. If this trend continues, and if duodenal ulcers are actually declining in frequency, as seems to be the case, there will be far less ulcer surgery in the future.

The type of operation that the surgeon chooses varies with his preference and experience. Most operations for duodenal ulcer do not actually remove the ulcer but deprive it of its acid sustenance, allowing it to "die on the vine," so to speak. There are several ways to accomplish this. The most common involves removal of the lower half of the stomach, which produces a hormone that stimulates acid. At the same time, the major nerves to the upper intestine may be severed, thus further eliminating a stimulus to acid secretion. This is called a *vagotomy*.

In another type of operation the stomach may be left intact, and only the nerves severed. A wider exit from the stomach is made at the same time, since the stomach becomes sluggish after its major nerves are severed.

A more refined approach to ulcer surgery has been gaining wider popularity. This involves carefully severing only those nerve fibers that stimulate the acid-producing portion of the stomach. This is called *highly selective* or *parietal cell vagotomy*. This operation holds great promise because the stomach is left largely undisturbed. Unfortunately, it cannot be performed in all instances of ulcer, and it requires some expertise.

No matter how effective surgery is, it cannot provide complete relief to every patient. The overwhelming majority of patients, however, can anticipate a very satisfying result.

WHAT ABOUT DIET?

This is usually the first question people ask after they have been told they have an ulcer. So firmly entrenched in most people's minds has the idea of a medical diet become that it has taken on the character of religious dogma. At times it seems to be just as zealously pursued. Of course, the medical profession itself must accept responsibility for this, ever since the Sippy milk and cream diet was introduced in the early part of this century and was as rigidly adhered to as if inscribed on the tablets on the Mount. Medical thinking about the role of diet in the treatment of ulcer disease has changed considerably in recent times. At present most experts believe that a person with an ulcer should be allowed to eat anything he wants, as long as it does not lead to distress. Most studies confirm that ulcer diets do not have much value. Unfortunately, popular medical myths die slowly, particularly those so all embracingly espoused by the medical community itself.

The fact remains, however, that most people with ulcers do quite well if they avoid those foods that cause symptoms, take proper medications and follow certain rules that still hold true:

1. Eat regularly and avoid long periods of fasting. Remember food itself is a buffer.

2. Find a substitute for coffee. There is probably some validity to the unfavorable reputation coffee has acquired among ulcer patients. It has been assumed for some time that decaffeinated coffee is a satisfactory substitute for regular coffee, because caffeine has long been known to stimulate stomach acid. Unfortunately decaffeinated coffee is just as potent as acid stimulus. While tea contains considerable caffeine, it seems to be better tolerated by ulcer patients.

3. Try to stop smoking. Cigarette smoking has been shown to adversely affect the healing of ulcers.

4. Must we avoid alcohol? There is no clear rule about

this. It is certainly prudent to abstain during an active flare-up, but the moderate use of alcohol with meals after the ulcer has healed has not been shown to increase the risk of igniting the ulcer.

5. Keep away from aspirin! Don't take advertised pain relievers that fail to state what they contain. Check the label to be sure. Aspirin probably causes more ulcers to bleed than any other medication.

6. Not all ulcer patients are high-strung or nervous. Emotional turmoil or conflict may produce stomach pain and distress. But it seems doubtful that emotional stress causes an ulcer. Tranquilizers should not be part of the long-term treatment of ulcers. They may be useful for a short time for flare-ups accompanying an emotional crisis. But they should not be used for long periods of time. After all, peptic ulcer is a lifelong problem and it is wiser to change life-styles and attitudes than attempt to use drugs to deal with symptoms.

LIVER AND GALL BLADDER TROUBLE

The gall bladder itself isn't impressive looking for all the trouble it causes. It is a lemon-sized, greenish structure located in the right upper part of the abdomen, hugging the liver and lying just beneath the rib cage (see Fig. 17). It stores bile made by the liver, releasing it on demand during meals.

Very often an abnormal gall bladder causes no symptoms at all. But sometimes it acts up, causing anything from vague indigestion to severe pain. The most typical pain is "boring" in nature—under the right rib cage, often shooting back between the shoulder blades and appearing after fatty or greasy meals. Contrary to what many people believe, discomfort after a fatty meal does not automatically indicate a gall bladder problem.

DIAGNOSING A GALL BLADDER PROBLEM

Gall bladder problems almost always begin with gallstones. These are typically dark and pearl-shaped but vary from tiny sandlike particles to large walnut-sized nuggets. It is surprising how often gallstones can be present without calling attention to themselves. These are referred to as *silent stones*.

How can your physician determine with certainty that a gall bladder problem exists in someone with abdominal distress? Fortunately, a number of reliable tests are available to trace the problem to the gall bladder. The most useful of these is the gall bladder series, which involves nothing more than swallowing a few pills of a special dye and taking an ordinary X-ray the next day to determine whether the dye has concentrated in the gall bladder. In most cases, gallstones will be picked up quite easily. If no dye appears in the gall bladder, the test may be repeated. If still no dye is found, this usually indicates an abnormal gall bladder.

A simpler and equally sensitive test for gallstones is called *ultrasound*. A small instrument emitting high-frequency sound waves is placed on the abdomen and through images created by the reflected waves, the gall bladder and other intra-abdominal organs can be clearly seen. The test is comfortable and very accurate, showing the presence of gallstones even an X-ray fails to show.

WHAT TO DO ABOUT GALLSTONES

Surgery is still the only permanently effective treatment for gallstones and a diseased gall bladder. Later in the chapter we shall discuss the newer approaches, including medicines to dissolve gallstones.

Sometimes the decision to operate is relatively easy. If the gall bladder becomes inflamed and swollen, resulting in severe pain and fever, a condition referred to as *acute cholecystitis*, most authorities agree that it should be removed. Even if the attack subsides, there is a high likelihood of recurrence with potentially serious complications. Likewise, there seems little alternative to surgery in cases of recurrent inflammation of the pancreas, or *pancreatitis*, associated with gallstones.

Blockage of the bile duct by gallstones has up until now been considered the clearest reason for surgery. The bile duct is a short rubbery tube that carries bile from the liver to the gall bladder and the intestines (see Fig. 19). Sometimes gallstones, which generally form in the gall bladder, are swept along with the current of bile. If they are too large, they may be unable to pass the narrow channel and instead lodge within the bile duct. This can dam the current of bile behind the stone and lead to jaundice and infection. Currently, it is felt that if the gall bladder is diseased, and the person is otherwise in reasonable health, it is wise to operate and remove the gall bladder, and simultaneously remove the blockage of the duct.

An alternative approach to direct surgery has recently evolved to dislodge stones caught in the bile duct. It involves a highly sophisticated technique by a skilled specialist using an optical instrument that the patient swallows. A cutting wire is inserted through the instrument and directed to the tiny opening where the bile duct enters the bowel. By means of an electrical current, this pinhead-sized aperture is widened to allow the large stones entry into the bowel. There are only a handful of specialists skilled in this technique at present, and it is still unclear which patients are the best candidates. Most specialists agree that the person in poor health who has had his gall bladder removed previously and develops blockage by a stone is the most obvious candidate. Opinions remain divided about whether anyone with stones caught in the bile duct should have this procedure first, especially if a gall bladder filled with stones is left behind. Surgery is still favored for someone in reasonable health.

Why the concern about stones in the bile duct? Bile stagnating behind a stone damming the current of bile can lead to jaundice, ill health, and liver damage. More importantly, it sets the stage for life-threatening infections. Inflammation of the pancreas is another of the potentially serious consequences.

SILENT STONES

Sometimes gallstones are found accidentally during investigation of another problem or in someone with other very minor complaints. These are called *silent stones*. Here there is room for disagreement about what is best to be done. Studies show that about half of the people with silent stones will eventually run into difficulty. For this reason, current medical belief is that people under sixty will best benefit from gall bladder surgery, largely because they face a very small risk from the surgery. On the other hand, any decision based exclusively and arbitrarily on age is not rational. Certainly there are many people in their sixties and seventies who are in better health than their younger friends. Moreover, the doctor must be free to take into account just how severe the individual symptoms are, that is, just how "silent" those stones are. At present, most doctors are inclined to treat older people with cautious care—resorting to surgery only when it is absolutely necessary.

DISSOLVING GALLSTONES

A flurry of excitement both in medical and lay circles has greeted the recent demonstration that certain gallstones can be dissolved by bile salts taken by mouth. At this writing, national trials have just been completed to assess the overall efficiency and safety of this novel approach. It has already been shown that these medications can shrink and dissolve stones very dramatically in selected patients. Certain limitations of this treatment have already become apparent and it is clear that not everyone will benefit from it, particularly those whose gallstones are heavily calcified or whose gall bladder cannot be seen on a gall bladder X-ray. Furthermore, not all stones dissolve completely and many seem to reappear after the medicine is stopped. Since use of the drug is still in the early stage, we need more information before we know who can benefit most from it. If, as it seems, the drug must be used for a lifetime, it is doubtful that it is suitable for younger patients.

JAUNDICE

While the jaundiced patient may not hold a "jaundiced" view of life, he certainly has reason to be upset. The yellow skin and yellow eyes of jaundice are not just a cosmetic problem. The underlying cause of jaundice, a liver problem, is a reason for concern. In the younger person, jaundice usually results from an inflammation of the liver, or *hepatitis*. While the same may hold for the older person, much more often the problem lies in a blockage of the bile duct.

Because people with jaundice frequently feel well, they may tend to dismiss it and delay a visit to the doctor. *Jaundice always means that a problem exists!* Never postpone a checkup if you notice that your eyes or skin have turned yellow.

Jaundice is commonly a result of a blockage of the bile duct by a gallstone or tumor. Other problems, however, such as hepatitis or other liver inflammation, can lead to jaundice. Many of the drugs that are taken by older people can produce jaundice. Very rarely, certain types of anemia that destroy blood cells can also cause mild jaundice.

The problem confronting your doctor when you come to him with jaundice is to discover the exact cause. Fortunately, several newer techniques now allow us to investigate the bile ducts to see if they are clogged. We have alluded to these techniques previously as *ultrasound* and *ERCP* (see page 119). This latter procedure involves swallowing a fiberoptic instrument through which a small tube is passed into the opening of the bile duct in the intestine. Dye can then be injected into the bile duct or the pancreatic duct (see Fig. 19). Another simple technique involves passing a very thin needle, called, appropriately enough, *skinny needle*, through the skin of the abdomen into the liver, which punctures a small bile duct so that dye can be injected. Some institutions have access to a highly sophisticated machine called the whole-body CAT scanner, (see page 118) which can often determine whether there is blockage to the bile ducts.

With the available techniques, it is possible in most cases to decide whether the jaundice results from an obstructed bile duct. If no obstruction is found, it may be necessary to examine a small piece of liver tissue (liver biopsy). This is easily obtained in a matter of seconds with a small needle inserted through the skin into the liver. Such problems as inflammation of the liver or scarring of the liver, called *cirrhosis*, can be easily diagnosed by examining the tissue. And you don't have to be a drinker to get cirrhosis! Many people are upset when they have been told they have cirrhosis, particularly those who have never taken alcohol. They are obviously victims of a popular misconception. There are, in fact, many causes for scarring of the liver. Sometimes doctors are unable to identify the cause. In any event there is no specific treatment for the scarring. Your doctor will recommend certain changes in diet, as necessary for your condition.

If the condition has been present for some time and the biopsy shows inflammation of a chronic nature (*chronic active hepatitis*), it may be necessary to take cortisone to control the condition.

Jaundice is not a simple condition. Don't expect your doctor to come up with an immediate answer. It is true that sometimes a few blood tests will promptly pinpoint the problem, but don't count on it. Usually it takes a systematic, well-reasoned approach to uncover the real cause of jaundice.

SUMMARY

1. Digestive complaints are common as we grow older. Minor unchanging complaints over a long period of time should not be a cause for undue concern. Common-sense measures will usually control most symptoms. When new symptoms occur or worsen medical help should be sought. A number of newer diagnostic techniques permit more accurate diagnosis of digestive complaints than ever before.

2. Heartburn is usually due to acid backflow from the stomach. There are simple measures to control these complaints and only rarely will surgery be required.

3. The sense of food sticking in the chest after eating is always a serious symptom and should be investigated.

4. Ulcers cannot exist without acid and therefore the treatment involves eliminating the acid. Any food buffers, acid and dietary restrictions have little value in themselves. Aspirin, cigarettes, alcohol, and coffee may aggravate ulcers and should be avoided. Newer medications are available for treatment.

5. Most gallstones do not cause problems. Surgery is required only for gallstones that cause serious symptoms. Newer methods to dissolve gallstones will probably benefit only a selected number of people.

9

THE DISCONTENTED
BOWEL

Each day our media assure us with numbing repetition that
health and contentment are the rewards of "regularity."
Older people are particularly vulnerable to these advertise-
ments, since bowel habits are more likely to change with the
passing years. The almost irresistible lure of clockwork "regularity" often creates needless anxiety in older people and
convinces them that something serious exists if they are
unable to achieve this.

It is unfortunate that so much false and misleading information has grown up about what a "normal" bowel movement means. Actually, we have no precise definition of a
normal bowel movement. It varies from person to person.
One individual may have a bowel movement every day, another every other day, and still another twice a day. Yet all
are experiencing normal bowel movements.

As you grow older there is a natural tendency for your
bowels to grow more sluggish. In most people this is simply
a result of natural changes in diet and reduced physical activity. It is therefore unreasonable to continue to expect
punctuality from your bowel. This expectation often creates
a sense of desperation in some older people, causing them to

pay excessive attention to the way their bowels are functioning. When you were younger, nature's call for bowel evacuation was a momentary incident, a casual ritual observed but unnoticed in the flurry of the day's activities. As you grow older, there are fewer distractions and more time to dwell on what were previously just minor occurrences. And then, of course, there are those laxative commercials, warning of dire events to come, if you do not begin your day with a regular bowel movement.

We do not wish to minimize the importance of some regular bowel movement pattern. What we do want to emphasize, however, is that each person has his own particular pattern and that this may undergo some minor modification with age.

HOW YOUR BOWELS WORK

Most of the food you eat is broken down and absorbed before it reaches the lower part of your intestines, which is called the *large bowel* or *colon* (fig. 23). This is the last segment of the long digestive tube where undigested food remnants are further decomposed, compacted, and stored until the signal is given to get rid of them. Stool is moved along and evacuated by a gentle kneading movement of the bowel. Stool will change in consistency, size, or shape according to the amount of water that it contains, the types of foods you have eaten, and the degree of squeezing movement your bowel exerts at the time of evacuation.

REPORTING YOUR BOWEL PROBLEM

Perhaps because of wide media discussion, most people will readily discuss their bowel problems with their physicians. Yet when these same people are questioned for an accurate description of their bowel movement, the doctor often finds them embarrassed and hesitant. Yet, as we shall see, it is most important to be aware of the appearance of the bowel movement. It is particularly important to be alert to the presence of blood in the stool. On the other hand, the unwritten proscription against observing one's own bowel movement often leads to needless anxiety in people who have noticed some changes in their stool and are shy about reporting it to their doctors. In fact, most changes that occur in the appearance of stool have a simple explanation and seldom imply a serious problem.

KINDS OF BOWEL PROBLEMS

There are many different bowel problems you may encounter as you grow older. Most are insignificant. A few are more serious. Among the complaints that people commonly report are:

1. Change in the appearance of the stool
2. Discomfort during a bowel movement
3. Change in the frequency of bowel movement
4. Blood in the stool.

1. CHANGE IN THE APPEARANCE OF STOOL

Stool is composed of the residue of food we have eaten, mixed with water and the bacteria that normally reside in our lower intestine. Although only the undigestible portion of what we eat remains, the residue nevertheless is a reflection of the kinds of food we eat, both in its consistency and its color. For example, a reddish color may be imparted by large amounts of red beets. A very light color may occur in people who eat predominantly dairy products. Iron pills and medicines containing bismuth (Pepto Bismol) impart a dark or even black color to the stool. These are unimportant. On the other hand, the sudden appearance of a very black bowel movement must be taken seriously. Internal bleeding may cause the stool to become black and liquid—the so-called tarry stool. If you notice this kind of bowel movement, you must seek medical help immediately. A very pale-to-white stool—"clay colored"—could indicate some blockage in the liver. If your bowel movement remains persistently pale on a normal diet and you don't feel well, discuss this with your physician. If there is a liver problem, your skin and eyes will often turn yellow, which will alert you to the importance of the stool changes.

A change in the size or shape of the stool is one of the most common concerns of older people, but one that rarely merits the degree of uneasiness people develop after noticing it. Most commonly, patients report a number of small, hard, stonelike stools. These are usually caused by prolonged drying of the stool in the bowel and an abnormal kneading action of the intestine. This erratic squeezing movement of the bowel can also cause the stool to become thin and flat, ribbonlike. These are normal variations and seldom indicate a serious problem.

One change that may indicate a potentially more serious problem is a gradual decrease in the caliber of the stool: it becomes progressively thin, pencil-like. While this does not necessarily mean that something is seriously wrong, it is best to have your doctor check it. The appearance of blood in your stool always requires medical attention (see page 150).

Mucus with stool usually does not indicate a serious problem. If it occurs often and in large amounts, this should be checked, since on occasion certain types of polyps and inflammation of the bowel can cause this symptom.

2. DISCOMFORT DURING A BOWEL MOVEMENT

Any irritation in the rectal area will cause some pain during a bowel movement. Although the condition may be a very minor one, the pain can be quite intense. Most often a small tear, called a *fissure*, or a clotting hemorrhoid (*pile*) is to blame. Tiny infected tunnels called *fistulae* can stir up a great deal of discomfort because of their strategic location in this narrow area. However, more serious problems can exist. Don't try to treat them yourself. True, home remedies occasionally give some relief. But since they do not attack the cause of the problem, this can be dangerously misleading. Leave the diagnosis and treatment to your doctor.

A constant urge to have a bowel movement very often in the morning with a discomforting feeling of incomplete evacuation may indicate a more serious problem, particularly if it is a recent development. This should be reported to your doctor at the earliest opportunity.

3. CHANGE IN FREQUENCY OF BOWEL MOVEMENT

Our advertising media would have us believe that preserving the appearance of youth can somehow preserve the carefree spirit and vitality of youth. Hair dyes and dental adhesives may restore a more satisfying self-image but will not reverse normal biologic changes. Yet older people are quick to relate to those grim and weary TV figures who rebound with fresh vitality and bouncy exuberance after using the right laxative. After all, here is a simple explanation and remedy for their own normal fluctuations in well-being. In fact, this only perpetuates one more myth about bowel function and its effect on general health. Frequency of bowel movements has nothing to do with general well-being. Occasionally, though, you may have a significant and persistent change in frequency, which may require medical attention.

4. BLOOD IN THE STOOL

This problem is discussed later on page 150.

DIARRHEA

Diarrhea is a relatively uncommon complaint in older people. Most of the time an attack is short-lived due to a viral infection or dietary indiscretion. Prolonged diarrhea may suggest a more important bowel disturbance and should be reported to your doctor. Very often diarrhea will alternate with periods of constipation. This usually indicates a disruption of the normal squeezing action of the bowel, which is discussed at length in the section on diverticulosis (see page 145). A prolonged period of constipation culminating in frequent small watery bowel movements with the sensation of incomplete evacuation may indicate blockage by impacted stool and also requires medical attention. In fact, this feeling of constant urge to have a bowel movement with only meager evacuation usually means the presence of some irritation in the rectum and should never be ignored.

On the whole, most cases of diarrhea can be controlled by simple measures. Older people more often face the problem of constipation.

CONSTIPATION

Your body is in some ways like complex interlocking gears of a finely crafted clock. As one gear slows, so must all of the moving parts. Generally speaking, the less active you become and the more your total life-style changes, the more likely are your bowels to become sluggish. Despite what TV commercials may tell you, sluggish bowels do not lead to tiredness, moodiness, or lack of vitality. A missed bowel movement for a few days does not cause any ill effects. Older people find it difficult to surrender their long-held notion that debilitating toxins are somehow generated by putrescent material retained in their body. This is sheer folklore and without any scientific basis.

There seems to be just as much confusion over how to define constipation. Strictly speaking, constipation is fewer bowel movements over the same period of time. Individuals vary widely in bowel behavior when they become constipated. A person who all his life has had two bowel movements a day and suddenly finds that two days pass repeatedly without a movement is constipated. If this new pattern persists for several weeks, seek medical attention to be certain that no serious problem, such as an underactive thyroid or tumor of the bowel, exists. On the other hand, someone who has never experienced a daily bowel movement should be content with this pattern and not begin to grow concerned over it when he is older.

While we have emphasized the slowing of bowel activity with the passing years, it is important to realize that many people retain an unchanging bowel pattern throughout their lives. In fact, older people who continue with their regular diet and lead active lives seldom experience marked changes in bowel behavior.

CONSTIPATION AND DIVERTICULOSIS

Since constipation and diverticulosis are often found together in older people, it is understandable how one came to be regarded as the result of the other. Diverticuli are tiny pouches that erupt from the wall of the bowel much as bubbles protrude from the surface of a weakened rubber tire (fig. 23). They are usually discovered during an X-ray examination called a *barium enema*. Diverticulosis is the term used to describe the presence of these tiny outpockets. It is now believed that these diverticuli are not the cause of constipation. Rather both the diverticuli and the change in bowel habits seem to be the consequence of a bowel that has lost its normal squeezing ability. Normally, bowel contents are pushed along by a gentle kneading action. For reasons that are not understood, this well-coordinated process may be disrupted and two portions of the bowel may squeeze simultaneously, raising pressure in between them. A similar situation exists when the two ends of a rubber balloon are squeezed, causing the center part to billow. The diverticuli are tiny pouches that are forced through a weakened portion of the bowel wall by increased pressure.

Now, if the diverticuli really don't play any role in the bowel disturbance, why should there be any concern about them? Simply because these tiny blebs may become inflamed or burst. This leads to a condition called *diverticulitis*. When this happens, there will be severe pain, fever, and serious bowel difficulties. The term *diverticulosis* and *diverticulitis* are often used interchangeably by patients, and even some doctors. But they are actually two different con-

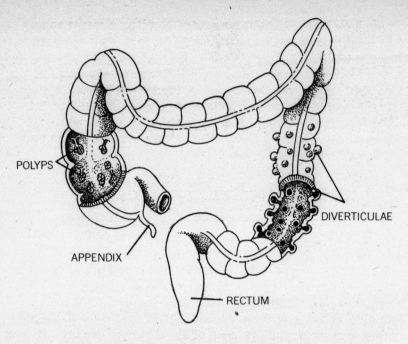

POLYPS

APPENDIX

DIVERTICULAE

RECTUM

Fig. 23   Large bowel (colon) showing polyps and diverticulae.

ditions. Diverticulosis simply indicates the presence of these tiny pouches, while diverticulitis is the condition that results when they become inflamed. Less commonly, a blood vessel near one of these pouches may bleed, causing the discharge of a large amount of blood through the rectum. This can be quite frightening. Although in some instances the bleeding may be great enough to require blood transfusions, in most cases it will stop by itself. Surprisingly, there is usually no pain present while this is happening.

Most patients with diverticulosis have no symptoms whatsoever. When there are bowel irregularities, the condition is often referred to as *diverticular disease* to emphasize the presence of symptoms. The bowel irregularities may vary widely. Some people are persistently constipated while others experience periods of constipation followed by periods of diarrhea. Diarrhea may even be the most constant complaint. Crampy pains, particularly in the lower left side of the abdomen, frequently accompany the bowel irregularity. There may even be a quiescent interval of normal bowel movements between periods of irregularity. Physicians often use the term *irritable bowel syndrome* to explain these symptoms when no bowel abnormality can be found. Since the condition closely resembles diverticular disease, treatment is similar for both conditions. An anticholinergic-type medication to relieve spasm is often used in the treatment of the irritable bowel syndrome.

The treatment of most forms of constipation whether or not diverticulosis is present requires an adjustment in diet. An essential part of this diet is the use of high-fiber foods.

HIGH-FIBER–HIGH-BULK DIET

There is very convincing evidence that our lower intestines actually require a certain amount of bulk to function at their best. This bulk is the residue it receives from the upper intestines and is composed mostly of the nondigestible portion of natural fruits and vegetables. This material, which remains undigested and eventually reaches the large bowel unchanged, is collectively called *fiber*. To most people the name seems to stir the mental image of some braided, ropy material making its knotty loops deep in their bowels and, so to speak, "tying things up." While this is a picturesque description, it does not tell us what is really happening.

There are in fact many different kinds of fiber composed of different chemical ingredients. What they have in common is that they are found in a wide variety of plants. All types of fiber resist digestion by the enzymes of the body. They thus reach the lower bowel virtually intact. A modern mythology has developed, centered on the miraculous properties of fiber or roughage and its ability to cure a variety of illnesses. It has not by means been proven that such a high-fiber diet will protect against heart attacks, gallstones, bowel cancer, and other afflictions claimed for it. Most of what we actually know about the effect of high-fiber diets is based on the fact that certain populations who consume a diet high in fiber suffer less from bowel disorders.

At present we really don't know the advantages of each of the many kinds of fiber. All, however, share one important property: They hold water within the bowel, thus making the stool swell and become bulky, somewhat the way a sponge soaks up water and swells.

Most people with bowel problems will benefit from the addition of fiber to their diet. Not too long ago, roughage or fiber was considered injurious to the bowel and many conditions were treated with a low roughage diet. Even the name "roughage" implied that these foods were harmful or irritating to the bowel. Now, fortunately, we know that just the reverse is true. The bowel actually requires a certain amount of bulk to help keep its tone just as our muscles require some active resistance to stay at their peak level. People with constipation due to sluggish bowels and people with diverticular disease will benefit from the addition of fiber to their diets.

Types of Fiber

What kind of fiber is best for people with bowel difficulties? There is no one, simple answer to this question, but we do know that almost any kind of fiber will exert some favorable effect. Although food fiber does differ in chemical makeup, it appears that the ability to hold water and swell is a common and most important property of all forms of fiber. The highest content of fiber will be found in grain products and foods high in grain content.

Bran, which is derived from the outer coat of the wheat kernel, contains the most fiber, almost 90 percent, and retains water best.

A rising interest in fiber has made readily available many food products containing high concentrations of bran, such as bread, muffins, and cereal. In addition, most stores now carry pure, unprocessed bran that can be mixed with prepared foods.

Many people, unfortunately, find the side effects of large amounts of bran as distressing as their bowel problems. Bloating, burping, gassiness, and abdominal cramps are not uncommon. For these people there are many alternative sources of fiber besides bran. Many fruits and vegetables are high in fiber. Apples, carrots, mangos, brussels sprouts, and corn meal contain substantial quantities of fiber with significant water-holding capacity. Lesser but still quite adequate amounts of fiber are found in peas, pears, oranges, green beans, and celery. In fact, all fruits and vegetables contain fiber. For the high-fiber diet to be most successful in the treatment of constipation, liberal amounts of fluid must be taken with meals.

TREATMENT OF CONSTIPATION

Although some slackening of bowel activity is common as you grow older, never assume that this is the reason for irregularity. Consult your doctor. If he agrees that there is no underlying medical problem, you can make a serious effort to regain some degree of bowel regularity. Most people will obtain some improvement by following a few simple rules, although in individual cases results will vary.

1. Try to keep to a daily routine. Choose a convenient time for a bowel movement when you won't be rushed or interrupted. For most people this is around breakfast time.

2. Begin with a gentle stimulus that can signal your bowel on a daily basis. A morning glass of prune juice, preferably cold, has earned a favorable reputation for just such purposes. On the other hand, some people find a morning cup of coffee just as suitable or even better. Cereal high in bran content can be started at this time and may prove effective even without additional stimulus. For most people with long-standing constipation, a more powerful stimulant to the bowel will usually be necessary for the first week or two. Any number of well-known cathartics are satisfactory. These can be taken on arising or at bedtime depending on the promptness of response. Some people find that a glycerine suppository or even stronger suppositories are necessary at the start. Enemas should be avoided until all else fails. Even then make every effort to discontinue enemas at the earliest moment.

3. Slowly increase the amount of bulk in your diet. In addition to breakfast cereals many products are high in fiber including breads and other baked goods. Vegetables and fresh fruit should be a regular part of your meals. If for some reason, you cannot tolerate adequate amounts, substitute products are available in the form of powdered vegetables or psyllium seeds. These provide the bulk your bowel requires.

4. Drink liberal amounts of fluids with meals and in between. Your doctor can recommend a mild stool softener that can be taken with a glass of water if stool remains too hard on fluid alone.

5. Keep active. Exercise is a vital part of any program for bowel regularity. A steady program of regular activity, even if this means only a short walk, improves bowel function.

6. Don't be discouraged if you fail to achieve that elusive daily movement. Be content if you have a reasonable pattern of regularity, even if it means missing a day or two, now and then.

BLOOD WITH A BOWEL MOVEMENT

Never ignore any bleeding that occurs with a bowel movement whether you notice it on the paper or in the bowl. Contact your doctor immediately. Let him decide whether this deserves serious attention. He'll probably order some tests, some of which may seem extensive for such a seemingly minor problem. But with blood in the stool it pays to be cautious. Even when you have had bleeding hemorrhoids for a long time, another condition may be responsible for the bleeding. This is especially true when the bleeding becomes more frequent or reappears after a long absence.

Even though in most people the bleeding will have a simple explanation, prompt attention may prevent serious consequences in those few people who do have a more significant problem. Minor conditions, such as hemorrhoids and fissure, frequently bleed. Diverticulosis will do so also, although more striking amounts of blood will be seen. Certain

abnormal blood vessels in the bowel may also bleed profusely. What we are really on the lookout for, however, are
polyps and tumors of the bowel.

POLYPS OF THE BOWEL

Very commonly, polyps of the bowel will reveal themselves by some small amount of blood with a bowel movement. Many lay people are justifiably confused about polyps
of the bowel and what should be done about them. Doctors
must share a great deal of the blame for this bewilderment.
For while much has been known about polyps for years,
authorities have differed among themselves on how to handle them. Recent developments, however, have helped to
simplify the problem.

A polyp is a growth from the wall of the bowel (see
Fig. 23). Some polyps grow like bushes from the wall of the
bowel, while others dangle from a long stem or stalk.

Polyps also differ in the type of cells that compose
them. For decades the polyp has been at the center of a
controversy concerning its relationship to cancer of the
bowel. Most authorities now believe that most bowel cancers begin as a polyp but that few polyps actually ever
become malignant. Current evidence indicates that the
chances of a polyp containing some cancer cells increases
directly with its size. Of course, judging the cancer risk of an
individual polyp isn't quite this simple, since other factors,
such as the appearance of the polyp and its constituent cells,
are also important. Nevertheless, most experts believe that
large polyps should be removed. This eliminates the need for
bothersome, frequent return visits and at the same time re-
moves a potential site for cancer. Small polyps are less a
cause for concern but many specialists now believe that they
too should be removed.

COLONOSCOPY

The colonoscope is a long, flexible tube that can be passed
through the rectum, permitting the doctor to directly view
the entire large bowel. Since it requires a great deal of ex-

pertise to perform a colonoscopy, only specialists in bowel diseases or other trained physicians will possess the necessary skills. Thorough bowel cleansing is required before this procedure can be performed.

With the colonoscope it is now possible to detect bowel problems up to now hidden to other means of investigation. Just as importantly it has revolutionized our attitudes about polyps of the bowel. Polyps deep in the bowel that previously required surgery can now be removed with instruments passed through this tube. Since this is a relatively simple procedure, most specialists remove even smaller polyps rather than take chances in the future. However, not all polyps can be removed by this method, and it may be necessary in some situations to perform an operation through the abdomen.

CANCER OF THE BOWEL

Intensive educational efforts by many health-minded groups have raised the general level of awareness of cancer as a national health problem. Sometimes it seems that the effort has been too successful. It has created a fear of cancer that too often becomes an obsession, a menacing companion stalking the patient who notices some change in his bowel movements. Most physicians sense the oppressive, unseen presence of this fear from the start. For the most part this is an unreasonable fear. The majority of bowel complaints are due to minor or insignificant problems. Keep this fact in mind should you develop a bowel problem. Moreover, cancer of the bowel is curable when caught early.

There is no one symptom of cancer. Diarrhea, constipation, blood with a bowel movement, or persistent abdominal cramps are some of the common warning signs. Any one of these symptoms that develops for the first time requires medical attention.

Cancer Checkup

Because cancer of the bowel becomes more common as people grow older, a sensible preventative approach should include a yearly visit to your doctor. With a simple test of your stool it is possible to detect blood that is not visible to the naked eye. This test can be done quickly after a rectal examination or on a stool specimen which you can bring or send in. *It is the simplest, most effective screening test for cancer of the bowel.* Your doctor will tell you how to prepare for it. He may also decide to examine your rectum with an instrument called a *proctoscope*. With this short tube he can check the lower end of your bowel. This procedure takes only a few minutes and causes only slight discomfort in most people. Most physicians now regard this test as an essential part of good routine health care.

Often it will be necessary to obtain more detailed information about the bowel. In such cases an X-ray called a *barium enema* will be necessary. This involves inserting a thick white material called barium through an enema tube while taking X-rays. The most precise examination however is colonscopy (see page 151). Because of its high degree of accuracy, physicians are increasingly relying on this procedure in cases where they feel the other tests do not provide sufficient information. Failure to find a source of blood in the stool in the large bowel requires additional investigation of the stomach and intestines with X-ray and endoscopic studies.

Because cancer of the bowel is so widely discussed, it is quite probable that you know someone suffering from this illness. Many are probably cured, while others sought help too late. Don't let irrational fears and unverified information deter you from seeking appropriate medical help when a problem develops. Even if you are in good health, have a yearly checkup. Many conditions can be picked up at a very early stage when simple measures may be able to take care of them.

SUMMARY

1. Nature never dictated that you must have a bowel movement every twenty-four hours. People's bowel habits vary considerably. What is normal for you is normal. Don't

feel that you have to conform to the pattern of other people's bowel habits.

2. You can develop reasonably regular bowel habits by following a balanced diet, drinking plenty of fluids, and exercising regularly and sensibly.

3. Never neglect a sudden and persistent change in your bowel habits.

4. If you see or suspect blood with a bowel movement, see your doctor immediately.

5. Polyps of the bowel are very common, but today they can usually be removed with reasonable safety without surgery.

6. Complete cure of cancer of the bowel is usually possible if diagnosed early.

10

FOOD
AND FADDISM

"We are what we eat." How often have you heard that old cliché? Certainly there is some truth in it.

Choice of food is one of the very few methods we have of regulating our bodily functions. But despite many decades of research, we have learned relatively little about nutrition in the past forty years. This does not restrain many self-appointed experts from issuing definitive statements about the values or dangers of various food substances. Writers, radio and television celebrities, health magazine editors, and even distinguished scientists outside of medicine have claimed to find in the foods we eat cures for—and causes of—cancer, arthritis, and many other maladies. Our purpose here is to explore what is known about nutrition, what is not known, and what food fads should be avoided.

OBESITY

The most prevalent and dangerous cause of malnutrition in the United States and in most other affluent nations is eating too much. We know now, beyond any doubt, that it is much healthier to be thin than fat. In fact, our normal standards for body weight have decreased over the last few decades. A person considered to be of normal weight at the turn of the century would be overweight by modern medical standards. Almost all the health statistics that we have amassed seem to favor the thin person. Thin people tend to live longer, have less heart disease, fewer respiratory infections, less arthritis, more stamina, and a happier outlook on life.

Increased weight and fat tissue in the body cause damage in both obvious and subtle ways. It is easy to understand how the stress of holding up excessive weight leads to damage of the two major weight-bearing joints—the hips and knees. The result: Obese people in their fifties and sixties and occasionally even in their forties may begin to have the pain and discomfort of arthritis. In time, the joint surfaces rub against each other and get chipped so that standing and walking become very painful. After a while, the person may have difficulty in balancing himself and may even require a cane to walk.

People who are overweight often have breathing problems. The breathing muscles must work harder to expand their lungs and bring oxygen to the cells of their bodies. After a while, these muscles may tire, and the heavy individual cannot breathe deeply anymore. Shallow breathing makes you prone to pneumonia, influenza, and bronchitis. Bacteria and viruses become trapped in the lungs instead of being whisked out of the lungs by the flow of air.

Some fat people breathe very poorly, and their lungs expand very little. This causes accumulation of carbon dioxide in the blood and very low blood oxygen levels. These people become lethargic and sleepy and develop heart trouble. This is called the Pickwickian syndrome, so named after the fat boy exhibiting these symptoms in Charles Dickens' *Pickwick Papers*.

If an obese person feels lethargic and unhappy, part of this may be because his body is constantly working harder to carry his excess weight around. But above and beyond the physical problems that accompany obesity, the obese person carries around some pretty serious emotional ones, too. He knows he is considered physically unattractive. He is a source of embarrassment and frustration to his friends and relatives and an object of ridicule. To a fat person there is nothing funny about obesity.

FACTORS LEADING TO OBESITY

What causes obesity? We do not really know. But we are sure that being overweight is not merely a matter of self-indulgence or moral weakness. It is a real disease like any other disease. Obviously, the fat person consumes too many calories for the amount of physical activity he performs. What he does not use up is deposited in his body in the form of fat. But we all know some people who eat enormous amounts of food and remain thin while others must struggle throughout their lives to keep their weight down by perpetual dieting. Why the difference? We don't really know for sure. But fatness and thinness seem to run in some families.

The amount of physical activity also affects our weight. Thin and overweight people have different life-styles. Many obese people do not burn up calories rapidly because they do not expend a great deal of physical energy in their daily activities. Studies have shown that obese people tend to sit still, often move slowly, lack animation. The thin person on the other hand is in motion, even when he is sitting, talking, and often even while sleeping.

Why can't a heavy person stop eating? In many people, emotional factors are at the root of their overeating. Eating is often an outlet for a number of psychological problems. Some people eat out of frustration and discontent. Eating becomes a substitute source of satisfaction for people who feel a sense of emptiness in their lives. They crave food to replace sexual, social, or work satisfaction. Sometimes, they are insecure and use obesity as a shield to keep others away from them. Overeating may even be a self-destructive impulse in a guilt-ridden individual.

There is much that we do not know about the development of appetite patterns. But there is no question that eating habits can be learned. People who eat too much in infancy and childhood tend to be heavy as adults. Children exposed to a great deal of confectionery tend to have more of a craving for sweets throughout life than those who were not taught to like these foods.

At the base of the brain is an area called the hypothalamus that regulates a number of bodily functions including appetite. Animals can be made to starve themselves or overeat when various parts of the hypothalamus are injured. We have reason to believe that the hypothalamus plays an important role in appetite control of human beings, but we don't understand how it works.

Clearly, we must realize how complex a matter obesity is. We must not look at fat people as morally weak. Their problems are physiological, psychological, and hereditary. Generalizations in the field of obesity may be misleading and dangerous.

TREATMENT OF OBESITY

The list of "cures" for obesity is almost endless. Unfortunately, the results have been generally poor. Losing weight is hard work; keeping it off is even harder. Every effective program for weight loss relies primarily on a marked reduction in the number of calories we eat. There is no shortcut to weight loss. Increasing physical activity won't help if you don't eat less.

The best way to take off weight is to cut down on calories in a steady, moderate fashion. It is healthier to lose a few pounds per week over a long period than to go on a crash diet. To do this, you must develop a consistent pattern of eating. This requires mental discipline. You cannot afford temporary lapses. These quickly become permanent lapses. You must show restraint even at dinner parties or on special occasions until you have lost as much weight as you want to or need to lose.

It is important to have some measure of the calories that you consume. If you normally require 2,500 calories to maintain your weight, lowering your intake to 1,200 calories over a long period will allow you to lose weight at an easy, steady pace. Your diet should be nutritious and palatable. It should contain adequate protein (at least 1½ to 2 oz. of protein for a normal adult) and fruits and vegetables to prevent vitamin deficiencies. It should have enough choices so that your palate does not become bored. Some of the commercially available diets (such as Weight Watchers) are excellent.

The decision to diet more quickly depends on your general state of health and how overweight you are. If you are in good health, you can afford to lose weight somewhat more rapidly, particularly if your obesity is threatening your health. But for some people, this course can be quite dangerous. People with heart disease, for example, may suffer a heart attack if they lose weight too rapidly.

Fasting

A fairly popular method of weight loss for very fat people is total fasting (eating nothing at all). If you fast for two to three weeks, you may lose fifteen to twenty pounds. You can then continue this diet by fasting one day a week in order to lose more weight and keep it off. Although prolonged fasting may seem like a very formidable stress, it is not difficult. If you stop eating, the body begins to break down fat for energy. The breakdown products (ketone bodies) begin to accumulate and suppress appetite. By the end of three or four days, you tend to feel weak, but no longer hungry.

This method of dieting is only for healthy people under a physician's close supervision. We would advise it only for very obese people who have great difficulty in reducing the number of calories they consume every day. We would also advise against fasting for people over the age of sixty. In addition to its rigorousness, it has another disadvantage. When you starve yourself, you tend to break down proteins from your muscles. At the end of a long fast, your muscles may be quite weak and flabby.

High-Protein Diets

There are many ways to curb your appetite. Eating a high-protein diet is a safe and effective way to lose weight. Cal-

orie for calorie, protein quenches your appetite better than
fat or carbohydrate. There is only so much meat and fish
that you can eat without becoming very full. You can also
drink a great deal of noncaloric fluid that will add to the
bloated feeling. Once you feel bloated and full, you will tend
to eat less.

Dangerous Fads

Some methods for losing weight are downright dangerous.
Here are two of the most widely used ones:

1. *Diet pills*. These are very popular, but also very dangerous, especially for older people. They curb the appetite
and are all basically members of a group of drugs called
amphetamines. They are potentially toxic and sometimes
even fatal. Amphetamines stimulate both the brain and
heart. In stimulating the brain, they make you feel alert but
they also cause sleeplessness and anxiety. You may slowly
and imperceptibly become "hooked" on these pills. When
you stop using them, you may feel drowsy and depressed.
These pills also speed up the heart and even cause heart
attacks.

2. *Liquid protein diets*. These are perhaps the most
dangerous of them all. Eating only liquid protein mixtures,
you become full easily and so decrease the number of calories you consume. However, this form of diet can produce
blood clots and disturbances of the heart's rhythm that may
result in sudden death. We strongly advise against liquid
protein diets.

In short, obesity is a complicated problem. It is certainly the most prevalent nutritional disorder in the industrialized areas of the world. For those of us who have a
tendency to gain weight easily, it is important to consider
the following:

1. Obesity is a many-faceted medical problem.
2. Eat a well-balanced and consistent diet, and avoid
   binges and snacks between meals.
3. It is important for you to remain as thin as possible.

4. If you are overweight, try to lose the pounds slowly but surely (two to three pounds a week) with a well-balanced diet of known caloric content.

5. High-protein intake and drinking noncaloric fluids may help by filling you up.

6. Avoid fads and diet pills.

7. Consult a physician before embarking on very low caloric diets.

8. Psychotherapy may be helpful if an emotional problem has triggered your overeating.

IMPORTANCE OF FIBER IN THE DIET

For some time, we have been noticing an apparent relationship between what we eat and the diseases we suffer from. For example, in the industrialized and affluent nations, the amount of roughage (such as lettuce, cucumber, bran, and fruit skins) in the average diet has dropped drastically. Instead, people eat more refined and artificial foods. Among these same people, we also find an increase in constipation and cancer of the colon. Colon cancer has increased at an alarming rate in the United States and is attacking people at an earlier age. In many underdeveloped areas of Africa, the diet is still high in fiber content, bowel movements are soft, and colon cancer is rare.

We now think that the origin of cancer of the colon lies in the toxic chemicals in food or from the lining of the intestines, which may lead to cancerous changes in the cells of the colon's inner lining. If this is so, it is important for the bowel to eliminate these substances quickly. It is well known that there is a high correlation between constipation and colon cancer. Lack of roughage certainly produces harder stools. Harder stools mean less frequent bowel movements. Less frequent bowel movements mean that toxic substances may remain in the colon long enough to produce changes that may eventually lead to cancer.

Many experts now advise an increase in the roughage

content of our diets. An excellent form of roughage is fiber in the form of bran. A bowl of cereal with a high bran content each morning adds a great deal of roughage. Bowel movements quickly become softer. Unfortunately, some people cannot tolerate bran well and develop stomach upsets. So they must obtain their roughage through fruits and vegetables. Although the data are not absolutely conclusive yet, we would recommend bran to all who can tolerate it, especially people who suffer from chronic constipation.

HIGH-FAT DIETS

The diets of people in affluent nations characteristically are high in saturated (solid) fats. This may have two very harmful effects. High saturated fat diets speed up hardening of the arteries and lead to heart attacks and strokes (see page 15).

Unfortunately, there is also increasing evidence to suggest that high saturated fat content in the diet, just like low fiber content, slows bowel movements and makes one susceptible to cancer of the colon.

As a general health measure, we advise everyone to avoid eating large amounts of saturated fat. For example: 1) Use skimmed milk and cheese products rather than whole-milk products. 2) Limit your intake of eggs and beef. 3) Eat poultry and fish instead of beef. 4) Avoid cooking with solid fats. 5) Do not deep-fry your food because this process converts unsaturated cooking oils to saturated fats. 6) When you do eat beef, have it on the well-done side.

UNDERNUTRITION

Despite the affluence of our society, many of our people do not eat enough food or the right foods. They are undernourished and suffer from specific dietary deficiencies. For a variety of social, economic, and medical reasons, elderly people fall into this group.

To begin with, their incomes are all too often inadequate. Retired people on fixed pensions find that inflation has seriously affected their purchasing power. Food prices have skyrocketed so that even most middle-class families must be careful in shopping to plan meals that are both nutritious and affordable. This means avoiding a lot of ready-made foods, stocking up on certain items when their price is temporarily lower, and cooking large quantities of foods that can feed several people for a relatively low cost per person. Unfortunately, older people may not always be able to follow these suggestions. Cooking for one or two people rather than four or five costs more per person. Quite often, older people don't have cars of their own or can't get transportation to a supermarket where they could buy large quantities of food less expensively.

Some single people, especially men, may not know much about cooking and may thus be forced to buy ready-made foods such as canned soups, TV dinners, and canned vegetables. This kind of diet is not only expensive but often contains foods that aggravate the common ailments of older people.

Many older people have lost their teeth and are wearing poorly fitting dentures. So they may have to live largely on liquids and soft foods. If they are depressed or easily confused and living alone, they may not be able to cope with the chore of preparing a meal. Ready-made foods of poor nutritive value thus may become the mainstays of their diet.

Under these circumstances, many older people are consuming foods lacking protein. They become frail. They lose their ambition and zest for living. Their mental processes slow up. Without protein, they cannot maintain their muscle strength or keep their vital organs functioning properly. If the blood protein level falls, fluid may escape from their blood vessels into the surrounding tissues. These people look swollen, puffy, and wasted. They may not realize how wasted they are because their weight may not have changed much. Fluid takes the place of muscle on the scale.

VITAMINS

In the early days of this century, some classical experiments established the essential roles of certain vitamins in maintaining health. One of the great sagas in the history of medicine involved the discovery of niacin. For many years lower-middle-class children in the southern United States developed a disease called *pellagra*. They would have bouts of severe diarrhea and bad skin rashes and would become lethargic and irritable. Surprisingly, the poorer Southerner rarely had this problem. After comparing the environment and diet of these two groups very carefully, public health officials noted a major difference in the quality of grains that these people consumed as major dietary staples. The poorer people ate coarse grains while the slightly more affluent were able to buy rice and other grains after they had been refined.

To carry the investigations further, the U.S. Public Health Service set up a huge field trial. With the help of prisoner volunteers, it was demonstrated that a diet consisting primarily of polished grains led to pellagra and substitution of unpolished (coarse) grains resulted in its cure. Later, people realized that niacin was present in the rough grains and lost when the grain was refined.

Other work led to the understanding of the relationship of other vitamins to important bodily functions. The following is a list of the major essential vitamins and their functions:

Vitamin A—is needed for healthy skin, eyes, and bones. A deficiency causes night blindness.

Vitamin B_1 (thiamine)—is needed for proper functioning of the heart and nerves.

Vitamin B_2 (riboflavin)—is needed for healthy skin and eyes. Deficiency may lead to skin ulcers and damage to the cornea.

Vitamin B_6 (pyridoxine)—is needed for proper functioning of nerves.

Niacin—prevents pellagra.

Folic acid—prevents anemia.

Vitamin B_{12}—prevents anemia and damage to the brain and spinal cord.

Vitamin C—prevents scurvy, a disorder that leads to bleeding gums, bleeding in the joints, and deformities of the bones.

Vitamin D—prevents rickets in children and osteomalacia in adults. In both these diseases, the body cannot place enough calcium into bones, and the bones become weak and deformed.

VITAMIN AND MINERAL DEFICIENCY

Malnutrition in the elderly may lead to vitamin deficiency. If an individual is deprived of fruits and vegetables, he may not be receiving adequate quantities of folic acid. We will point out in a later chapter (see page 201) that many older people develop anemia because of this deficiency. This is the most common vitamin deficiency in older people.

Occasionally, an older person may also become deficient in thiamine (vitamin B_1). If his heart is affected, he may suffer from shortness of breath and increasing swelling of the legs. Thiamine deficiency also leads to mental confusion, lapses in memory, double vision, and numbness of the feet. Addition of thiamine to the diet reverses most of these symptoms, but the memory damage may be permanent.

Of great importance in our diet is the mineral calcium. Many studies show that many Americans do not take in enough calcium throughout most of their adult lives. This deficiency predisposes them to softening of their bones (*osteoporosis*) (see page 228) as they grow older. Osteoporosis, most common in women after menopause, may cause a great deal of pain and discomfort as well as fractures. Therefore, all of us and particularly women should make sure that we maintain an adequate calcium intake throughout our lives. Two glasses of skimmed milk per day can provide this calcium.

NORMAL DAILY REQUIREMENTS

There are a few kinds of foods that we should all eat every day. The following brief guide can help you select a menu that will include these essential items:

1. *Protein*. Protein is essential for healing, renewal, and general health of body tissues. Good sources of protein include milk, egg whites, meat, poultry, fish, wheat germ, and soy protein. Beans, peas, peanuts, and cereal grains also supply protein, but this protein is not used as efficiently.

If one glass of milk, one egg, or one ounce of meat, fish, wheat or soy protein equals one protein unit, a 120-pound individual requires 7 units, and a 160-pound individual requires 9 units. More than 9 units are not needed, even if you weigh more than 160 pounds. Such a diet for one day could include, for example, 1 egg, ½-ounce wheat germ or cereal, 2 ounces of tuna fish, 1 glass of skim milk, and 1 chicken breast (3 oz.) for a total of 7½ units. Most foods made with flour and other grains also contain protein, so that the total will always be higher.

2. *Fluid*. Fluid is present in many fruits and vegetables, and in sauces and desserts. In addition, four glasses of fluid daily are recommended.

3. *Fiber*. Although fiber is not an essential element of the diet, we have previously pointed out its usefulness in aiding bowel function. Foods that are high in fiber include bran, peas and beans, apples, pears, and berries with skin, potatoes and rye and whole-wheat breads and cereals.

4. *Calcium*. At least two servings of milk or cheese are recommended. Many other foods, including some fish and green leafy vegetables, also contain calcium. Bakery products often have calcium added to retard spoilage.

5. *Vitamin A*. One helping of a yellow vegetable or fruit will supply this vitamin.

6. *Vitamin D* is made in skin which is exposed to sunlight. If you spend most of your time indoors, Vitamin D can be obtained from one glass of skimmed milk.

7. *The B vitamins (riboflavin, niacin, and thiamine)* are found in all of the foods listed in the section on protein, and in most vegetables and fruits.

8. *Vitamin C* can be obtained from a helping of citrus fruit or fresh tomato.

9. *Folic acid* is present in most fruits and vegetables but is destroyed by prolonged cooking. Therefore, vegetables should not be cooked until mushy. If you have trouble chewing firm vegetables, chop or blenderize them.

10. Most of the other vitamins and supplements (vitamin E, pentothenic acid, biotin, lecithin, vitamins B_6, B_{12}, and K) are either present in a great variety of foods or manufactured within the body by intestinal action.

As you can see from this guide, you do not need vitamin supplements if you eat a well-balanced diet. If, however, you are on a rigorous weight reduction program or do not have access to foods such as fruits, vegetables, and milk, a daily multivitamin pill may be advisable.

VITAMIN FADS

What about some of the other vitamins and assorted products that we see advertised? Are they worth taking? Thousands of people take large doses of vitamins C and E and so-called megavitamins every day. Vitamin C first became popular when Linus Pauling, a Nobel Laureate scientist, wrote a book claiming that this vitamin in high doses can prevent and cure the common cold. He quoted a number of medical studies reporting favorable results, but other people found that vitamin C had no effect on colds.

It is difficult to design an experiment to test for a relationship between vitamin C and colds. Many different viruses cause colds, and people exhibit natural differences in their susceptibility to these viruses. Also some people are more likely to be exposed to these viruses than others. At present, we have no real evidence to support Dr. Pauling's claim.

There are also claims that vitamins C and E and perhaps others may help to prevent cancer. Some investigators believe that vitamin C in high doses can block the development of colon cancer. The data are only fragmentary and are particularly difficult to interpret because we know so little about the basic causes of cancer. Surveys comparing the incidence of cancer in people taking and not taking various vitamins might eventually tell us whether they have any anticancer value. At present, we just do not know.

Other claims have been made for vitamin E. There are those who believe that this substance is a veritable fountain of youth. Some magazines claim that it can increase longevity, prevent arteriosclerosis, and improve sexuality. There is no evidence in human beings to support any of these claims. In fact, we know virtually nothing about the role of vitamin E in normal body metabolism or whether it is essential for good health. There are some studies in lower animals, however, that suggest a role for vitamin E in slowing down the aging process. But we need to know much more than we now know before we can intelligently recommend the use of vitamin E.

HIGH-SALT DIETS

Many older people live essentially on canned foods such as soup, tuna fish, and various packaged crackers. All of these items have a very high salt content. If the individual has some heart disease, this salt load may lead to serious symptoms. Fluid accumulates in the body, and a sick heart cannot pump this fluid to the kidneys. As a result, the fluid accumulates in the lungs and the person may become increasingly short of breath especially when lying in bed at night.

If your doctor tells you to restrict your salt intake, you must throw away your salt shaker and add no salt to food during or after its preparation. Highly salted foods, such as smoked meats and fishes, canned soups, salted crackers, pickles and similar condiments, and various sauces, are out.

SUMMARY

1. Try to stay on the thin side. It is much healthier for your heart, lungs, and joints to be a little underweight than overweight.

2. Try to keep your diet relatively low in saturated fat. This is particularly important for younger and middle-aged people.

3. Roughage in your diet is good for your bowels. Fiber products are a particularly good source of roughage.

4. Avoid fads of unproven effectiveness or safety.

5. If you require a special regimen such as a low salt or diabetic diet, make sure that you understand it completely so that you can adhere to it closely. Ask your physician to go over it with you in great detail. You must know the relative salt intake of everything you eat if you are on a low salt diet. A diabetic diet must spell out in detail an exchange system by which so much of one food item can be substituted for so much of another.

6. Avoid deep frying.

7. Above all, eat a well-balanced diet that includes protein, fresh fruits, and vegetables.

11

KIDNEY AND BLADDER AILMENTS

Unless we have a problem, most of us do not think much about how our urine is formed and eliminated. The urinary system does not impress us as much as organs like the heart and lungs. We are made more aware of the remarkably complex functions of these other organs by the constant reminder in the press and by our own experiences with "what happens when something goes wrong with these organs" or "when they don't work as they should." Serious kidney and bladder problems are fortunately much less common. Nevertheless, the process of removing waste from our bodies is an extremely complicated and precise system—an engineering marvel that cannot be duplicated anywhere. As we age, this waste removal system develops problems.

HOW THE NORMAL URINARY SYSTEM WORKS

Our two kidneys are situated, one on each side, deep in the abdominal cavity. They have the job of filtering the waste products from the blood and eliminating them from the body. Blood comes to the kidneys in the same way as it does everywhere else, through an artery and its branches, ending up in tiny vessels called capillaries. The walls of these kidney capillaries are porous and allow fluid to filter into the pipes (tubes) of the kidneys in much the same way that water seeps through a coffee filter. It consists of water, minerals, and waste products, principally urea and creatinine.

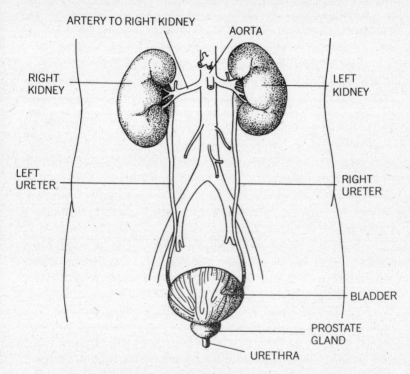

Fig. 24 Normal urinary tract. Note that the prostate gland surrounds the urethra where it leaves the bladder.

Urea is a nitrogen compound that is formed when the body uses protein for energy. Our bodies need only a certain amount of protein for building and repairing their cells. Excess protein is turned into urea, and fat and carbohydrate, which are stored in the liver for reserve energy. Creatinine is the waste product from our muscles.

The fluid filtering into the kidney pipes also contains many minerals and particles such as sodium, potassium, calcium, phosphate, chloride, bicarbonate and hydrogen. Blood proteins are too big to pass into the kidneys' tubes under normal conditions.

Under normal conditions, about 175 quarts of fluid are filtered from the bloodstream into our kidney tubes every twenty-four hours, and only one to two quarts actually leave the body as urine. If not for this remarkable ability of the kidneys to preserve fluid and bring it back to the bloodstream, we would not be able to survive for even a day.

The kidney tubes are remarkably selective. They can add to and subtract from the fluid that they receive from the bloodstream. Not only do the kidney tubes bring 173 quarts of fluid back into the bloodstream, but they also manage to bring back just the right amounts of each mineral. So the concentration in our blood of sodium, potassium, calcium, and other materials remains pretty normal no matter what our diet. For example, if the blood is too acidic but has too little sodium, the kidneys can make an exchange, bringing sodium from urine to blood and hydrogen (acid) from blood to urine.

After the urine leaves the kidneys, it goes through long narrow tubes called ureters (see Fig. 24). The ureters from each kidney meet in the bladder, located in the lower abdomen. The bladder is a muscular sac that stores the urine until we are ready to urinate. The bladder is kept closed by a muscle called a sphincter, which we can control up to a point. When it is time to urinate, the sphincter relaxes, and the bladder muscle pushes the urine into a tube called the urethra, which takes it out of the body (see Fig. 24).

It is apparent from this brief description that the kidneys are more than just waste removers. They help control the fluid balance of the entire body and respond constantly to internal needs. If your body loses lots of fluid from vomiting, diarrhea, or sweating, your kidneys will allow very little water and salt to be eliminated. If you drink a lot of water, the kidneys will eliminate more water. These mechanisms are almost unbelievably efficient in young normal people. You can recognize these adaptations of the kidneys by looking at your own urine. Drink a lot and the color of your urine tends to look like water. Take a walk in the hot sun, and your urine may become deep yellow or even brownish.

AGING AND THE KIDNEYS

As we grow older, our kidneys lose some of their ability to regulate the flow of water and minerals. Starting at about the age of forty, our kidneys can filter about one and one-half quarts less per twenty-four hours with each year of advancing age. They also lose some ability to determine how much of each mineral is eliminated in the urine. They cannot conserve as much sodium and water as they did before. Under normal conditions, this decreased capacity is not significant, but it may be important in some circumstances. For example, an older person may become dehydrated more easily than a younger person. Older people, therefore, must make sure that they drink sufficient fluid and add enough salt to their food in hot weather. Persistent vomiting requires earlier medical attention in the elderly than in young people.

KIDNEY DISEASE

If you develop kidney disease, more serious problems may occur. If the kidneys don't function properly, they no longer serve as a protection against loss of body fluid. So sweating, diarrhea, vomiting, or inadequate drinking can dehydrate a person, lead to low blood pressure and fainting, and even threaten his life. He may die if not treated promptly. Thus, even a simple cold or flu can be a very serious matter for a person whose kidneys aren't working well.

People with poorly functioning kidneys tend to develop anemia. The kidneys normally manufacture a substance called erythropoietin, which causes the bone marrow to make red blood cells. When the kidneys are damaged, they cannot produce enough erythropoietin, and so fewer red blood cells are made.

As the kidney failure worsens, waste products build up to a high level in the blood, and the individual becomes weak and lethargic, sleeping during the day and lying awake at night. We do not know exactly what waste products are responsible for these changes. In very severe kidney failure, certain acids and minerals accumulate in the blood to dangerous levels. If these materials are not eliminated, the individual dies. Fortunately, kidney disease usually does not progress to these advanced stages.

CAUSES OF KIDNEY PROBLEMS

Kidney failure can be caused by:

1. A disease affecting the kidneys themselves
2. A disease blocking the blood from getting to the kidneys
3. A disease blocking the urine from leaving the kidneys.

There are many processes that can damage the kidneys directly. Most involve an inflammation of the first part of the tube system (glomerulus, see Fig. 24) where the blood is first filtered. These diseases are called *glomerulonephritis*. In some cases, the glomerulonephritis is part of a disease affecting many areas of the body; sometimes it is limited just to the kidneys. We do not yet understand clearly the causes of these diseases.

The earliest sign of these diseases, even before kidney failure occurs, is the presence of protein in the urine. Normally, there should be almost no protein in the urine. Fortunately, most people who have protein in their urine never develop severe kidney failure.

A second group of kidney diseases involves the end portions of the kidney tubing. This *interstitial nephritis* can be hereditary in some cases, caused by certain drugs in others, and of unknown cause in many cases. This kind of kidney failure is usually associated with little or no protein in the urine and tends to progress more slowly.

The kidneys will also fail to function properly if not enough blood reaches them. This can happen when the heart fails to pump properly. Therefore, decreased kidney function is often a clue to the presence of heart disease. In other cases, the heart pumps adequately, but there is not enough blood available to pump to the kidneys. Thus, a dehydrated person may develop kidney failure. Finally, if there is hardening of the arteries (arteriosclerosis), blockage of the arteries feeding the kidneys will keep sufficient blood from reaching the kidneys.

When there is blockage of urine flow, the kidneys will also fail to function properly. This blockage can occur at the level of the ureters, bladder, or even beyond the bladder (see Fig. 24). Obstruction to urine flow causes the urine to back up into the kidneys and puts pressure on their pipes. This pressure gradually damages the sensitive cells of these pipes, and the kidneys begin to fail.

There are some diseases that cause kidney failure by more than one mechanism. For example, people with diabetes mellitus (see page 108) may have kidney disease related to all three basic problems. Diabetic people may have disease of the kidneys themselves as well as arteriosclerosis and clogging of the kidneys' arteries. In addition, if they develop damage to nerves (peripheral neuropathy), their bladders may become paralyzed (neurogenic bladder), blocking the normal flow of urine.

KIDNEY TESTS

If you develop symptoms of weakness or sleeplessness or are urinating very little, have your doctor check your kidneys. First, blood tests will measure the amount of urea and creatinine in the blood and will tell your doctor whether your kidneys are functioning normally. Once your doctor finds an elevated urea or creatinine blood level, he must proceed systematically to find the cause because treatment depends very much on an accurate and precise diagnosis.

Next, your doctor will test a specimen of your urine, looking especially for protein. If there is protein in your urine, the chances are that you have one of the disorders that affects the kidneys directly. It is important to measure how concentrated the urine is (specific gravity). If the urine is concentrated, this suggests that you have lost considerable body fluid, perhaps from vomiting, diarrhea, or excessive sweating. Drinking more fluids is usually adequate. In severe dehydration it may be necessary to receive fluid by vein in the hospital.

Finally, your doctor will want to determine whether your problem is entirely in the kidneys or is caused by some obstruction to urine flow after it leaves the kidneys. A new procedure called *ultrasound* may help locate where the trouble is. For this test, high-frequency sound waves are passed through the body at the level of the kidneys, and a special receiver picks up those waves that are reflected back. The procedure is simple, safe, painless, and outlines the size and shape of each kidney. If obstruction to urine flow is present, the kidneys become distended, and the ultrasound will show large kidney shadows.

If the kidney shadows are large, your doctor may order an X-ray test called an intravenous pyelogram (IVP) to confirm the presence of obstruction. For this painless test, an X-ray dye is injected into an arm vein and X-rays of the abdomen are taken as the dye goes through the urinary system.

Sometimes, it may also be necessary to pass X-ray dye through a catheter into the bladder and up the ureters toward the kidneys. This test, called a *retrograde pyelogram*, will show the doctor just where the obstruction is. If kidney failure is due to obstruction, surgery is generally needed to correct the problem.

If your doctor finds the problem to be inside the kidneys, it may be necessary to obtain a tiny piece of kidney for microscopic examination through a needle inserted through the back. This biopsy may provide information essential for choosing the right medications to improve kidney function. In most cases, a biopsy is not necessary.

ARTIFICIAL KIDNEY

If your kidney failure is not too severe, your doctor may be able to manage it by simply increasing your fluid intake. However, severe kidney failure requires a procedure called *dialysis*. In most cases, this dialysis is performed with an artificial kidney machine, but it can also be done through a tube placed in the abdomen.

The artificial kidney represents one of the great achievements of modern medical science. Thousands of people annually embark on treatment with this machine. They would otherwise die within days or weeks. Now they can live on for many years. Most important, the quality of their lives is generally good. Many are able to live normal lives.

The dialysis machine acts like a kidney to remove waste products from the body. In order to be connected to the machine, you must have a simple operation with a local anesthetic. An artery and a vein under the skin of your forearm are connected, forming what is called a *fistula*. Each time you are painlessly hooked up to the machine, your blood flows continuously through the dialysis machine and comes back again through the same fistula.

If you have severe kidney failure, you need to have dialysis with the kidney machine two to three times a week for about three hours at a time. Most kidney patients in the United States receive their dialysis in a hospital or clinic two or three times a week. However, some patients in the United States and many more in other countries such as England have learned to treat themselves at home with relatively easy-to-use machines. This home dialysis enables people to lead completely normal lives.

PROSTATE TROUBLES

One of the most common medical problems of older men is the enlarging prostate gland. The prostate gland is a small structure that sits right under the bladder and surrounds the urethra (see Fig. 24). As urine goes from the bladder to the urethra, it must pass the prostate on the way to the penis. The normal function of the prostate is not fully understood. Since sperm must also pass through it, some experts believe that the prostate must have something to do with normal sexual function.

In all normal men, the prostate enlarges with age. As it enlarges, it compresses the urethra and tends to block the flow of urine. At the same time, it begins to push on the bottom of the bladder and stretch the muscle that normally keeps the bladder closed. As a result of these changes, most men in their sixties and often in their fifties begin to notice that they must urinate more often and that their urine stream comes more slowly. A man who has never had to get up at night to go to the bathroom may have to urinate once, twice, or even more often during the night.

If these are the only symptoms, no treatment is necessary. However, the obstruction may become more severe, and then it may interfere with the work of the kidneys. Even if this does not happen, you may find yourself urinating almost every hour. The blockage of urine may also lead to recurrent infections in the bladder and kidneys.

Your doctor can determine the size of your prostate by feeling it during a rectal examination and by obtaining an IVP (see page 176).

TREATING THE ENLARGED PROSTATE

Although the occurrence of these complications depends mostly on how much the prostate enlarges, there is one thing that you can do to protect yourself. If you are beginning to have symptoms of an enlarged or enlarging prostate, put yourself on a regular schedule of urination. If you urinate every four or five hours, this will protect your kidneys from the ill effects of the blockage. In addition, the bladder will not become distended with urine, and it may be able to push the urine past the blockage.

If urine blockage becomes very severe, the only cure is surgery. Most of the time, this operation can be performed directly through the penis under local anesthesia. It is called a *transurethral resection*. The results of this operation are excellent, and most men never need a second procedure. Sexual function is usually not diminished by this operation.

CANCER OF THE PROSTATE

The development of cancer cells in the prostate increases with age. In fact, most men over the age of eighty have some cancer cells in their prostates. Fortunately, these cells usually grow slowly and do not travel beyond the prostate. However, spread to other areas of the body occurs often enough to make cancer of the prostate the most common cancer problem in men.

It is very difficult to diagnose prostatic cancer before it spreads because it causes no symptoms in its early states. Careful rectal examination, performed annually, may enable the physician to find cancer of the prostate in an early stage. Then surgical removal of the prostate or local X-ray treatments may be effective. When it spreads, it often goes to the bones, and many men with prostatic cancer experience pain in the back or ribs as the first symptom. Unfortunately, cancer of the prostate is often discovered at a later stage by X-ray of the painful bones and a blood test called *acid phosphatase*. Acid phosphatase is a protein that the prostate makes, and its concentration in blood is elevated when cancer develops and spreads.

Fortunately, prostatic cancer often grows slowly even after it begins to spread, and many men can get along with it quite well for months and even years. Treatment is not necessary unless you develop symptoms such as bone pain, weakness, and weight loss. The first line of treatment is hormones. Since male hormones make the prostate grow and female hormones cause it to shrink, your doctor may recommend removal of your testicles and treatment with estrogen. If this therapy is not adequate, there are other drugs that directly attack the cancer cells.

Unfortunately, despite the slow-growing nature of prostatic cancer, it is still a very significant cause of disability and death in older men because it is so common. Scientists have been searching for a method to detect prostatic cancer before it spreads from the prostate itself. If the diagnosis can be made at that stage, surgical removal of the whole prostate can cure the problem. Within the last two years, a promising new test has surfaced that may be the screening test we have been looking for. By a special test using radioactive material, it may soon be possible to measure minute quantities of acid phosphatase in the blood. The test can pick up the amount that a prostatic cancer produces when it is still only a small group of cells within the gland. Many experts believe that mass screening with this blood test for men over the age of sixty may result in the saving of thousands of lives.

URINARY INFECTIONS

Infection of the kidneys and/or bladder is a very common problem that increases in frequency with age. In young people, urinary infection is basically a disease of women, but after the age of fifty-five men also develop this problem. It is estimated that perhaps 15 to 20 percent of people over the age of sixty-five develop some kind of urinary infection, but only a small number have any symptoms. Young women develop infection in their bladders after they begin to have sexual intercourse.

Men do not develop bladder infection unless there is some obstruction to flow in their urinary system. A few bacteria from the skin are constantly invading our urethras, and they can multiply very quickly if there is not rapid enough urine flow to whisk them out through the urethra. Thus, men do not have any infection until their prostates begin to enlarge and slow down the stream of urine.

The most common place where urinary infection occurs is the bladder (*cystitis*). Symptoms include frequent need to urinate and pain with a burning sensation during urination. When you have these symptoms, your physician can usually see white blood cells and bacteria in your urine under a microscope. He will then order a culture of your urine in order to determine which bacteria are present and how many there are. He will begin treatment with a generally effective antibiotic while awaiting the report of this culture.

Your physician may change the antibiotic if the infection does not respond quickly. Generally, treatment requires seven to ten days, although sometimes one or two large doses of antibiotic is sufficient. A second culture should be obtained after treatment to make sure that all the bacteria have been eradicated.

Kidney infection (*pyelonephritis*) is more serious and may make you feel quite sick—usually with fever, low back pain, and sometimes nausea and vomiting. Again, the treatment is antibiotic, but it must be begun quickly. Sometimes you may have to be hospitalized for a brief stay.

CONSEQUENCES OF KIDNEY INFECTION

For many years, doctors believed that repeated urinary infections commonly lead to serious and permanent kidney damage. Fortunately, this belief has not stood the test of time. It is now quite clear that repeated or chronic infection will not damage the kidneys unless there is an obstruction to urine flow. If you develop infection, your doctor should order kidney X-rays (IVP) to look for an obstruction. If none is present, no further tests are necessary.

Many people have chronic infections without symptoms. As long as your IVP is normal, you need not worry about this kind of infection. Your doctor may want to try once to treat this infection with a mild antibiotic. If this does not work, it is generally advisable to leave the situation alone. Treatment with stronger and more dangerous antibiotics may cause more harm than good. Treatment becomes necessary only if you develop symptoms.

KIDNEY STONES

These stones are formed by the accumulation of crystals of certain minerals that ordinarily are dissolved in the urine. When these crystals are not fully dissolved in the urine, they may form stones that get stuck either in the kidney tube system or in a ureter. This condition causes very severe lower back pain that may travel in waves down the abdomen to the groin. The pain caused by kidney stones (called renal or kidney colic) is one of mankind's most uncomfortable conditions and generally requires large doses of morphine or Demerol for relief. Severe nausea and vomiting occur with the pain. There is usually some blood in the urine.

If you should have an episode of kidney colic, your doctor will usually hospitalize you and treat you with intravenous fluids and pain-relieving medicine. Most often, the stone will pass through the ureter within a few days and be eliminated in the urine. Your doctor will want all your urine strained until your pain is gone so that the stone can be caught and chemically analyzed. Future treatment may depend on this analysis. Sometimes, the stone does not pass by itself. Then it must be removed by surgery.

Stone formation is quite common in middle-aged and older people. Most people who develop a stone will have only one attack. If you have more than one attack, your doctor will suggest preventive steps based on what the stones are made of. In all cases of kidney stones, fluid intake is very important. Anyone who has had this problem should drink more fluid, especially in hot weather.

Stones can be formed from a number of minerals such as calcium carbonate and calcium phosphate and a waste product called uric acid. Calcium stones are by far the most common. Most of the time, no reason can be found for calcium stones. However, there are a number of conditions that raise the calcium level in the blood and occasionally lead to calcium stones. Thus, a blood test to check your calcium level is important if you have had a calcium stone.

Uric acid tends to form stones when the urine is too acidic. Therefore, your doctor may ask you to take sodium bicarbonate pills three times a day and another drug at bedtime in order to prevent your urine from becoming acidic when you have uric acid stones. This treatment is very successful in preventing uric acid stones. If your blood level of uric acid is high, he may ask you to take a drug called allopurinol, which lowers the amount of this waste product in your blood.

SUMMARY

1. Our kidneys are remarkably efficient filters that eliminate waste products and regulate the concentration of vital minerals in our blood.

2. If you have kidney troubles, you may become weak and tired. Consult your doctor.

3. If you have kidney problems, your doctor must order some tests to determine the cause. Many causes are correctable.

4. Even if the cause is not correctable, you can still lead a normal life with treatment through an artificial kidney.

5. Older men may have difficulty in urinating when their prostates enlarge. If the enlarged prostate blocks urine flow, a simple procedure may be necessary to eliminate the obstruction.

6. Cancer of the prostate is the most common cancer in men but fortunately it usually does not spread through the body.

7. If you develop symptoms of kidney infection, such as pain on urinating and frequent need to urinate, consult your physician. In addition to treating you with an antibiotic, he will order a test to find out whether the infection is due to blockage of urine flow.

8. Older people must be very careful to drink sufficient fluids because their kidneys may not conserve fluid as well as they once did.

12

FOR WOMEN ONLY

Men and women share more or less equally in the physical changes that come with aging. However, some, in the very nature of things, are unique to women, simply because they alone bear and nurture children. The organs that fit women for these unique functions are, unfortunately, subject to a wide variety of disorders and diseases.

In its specialty of gynecology, the medical profession has long devoted itself to dealing with the complexity of women's medical problems. With aging, these problems take on somewhat different and more complicated forms.

No women of any age can afford not to have a periodic, routine gynecological checkup whether they have symptoms or not. Some serious problems don't exhibit any symptoms at first. A checkup may pick up these problems before they have gone too far. Every adult woman should have a pelvic examination at least once a year during which a cytology (Pap) smear should be obtained. Many gynecologists advise having a Pap smear every six months. A Pap smear can pick up cancer of the cervix when it is 100 percent curable. It also helps detect cancer from other parts of the female organ system. If all women followed this advice, thousands of lives would be spared every year.

THE MENSTRUAL CYCLE

No medical subject is more fraught with emotional overtones than a woman's menstrual cycle. From time immemorial, all kinds of symptoms and illnesses have been ascribed to changes in vaginal bleeding. It is easy to understand why. After all, this regular, self-limited bleeding is a remarkable physiologic event that sets the female apart from the male. Ancient peoples were in awe of this event, attributing mystical qualities to it, and, at the same time, recognizing its relationship to fertility. Generations of women have learned from their mothers about menstrual bleeding and its trials and tribulations. They have come to see it, on the one hand, as a sign of physical and sexual maturity and potency and, on the other hand, as their weak and vulnerable time.

Hormones are the key factors controlling a woman's menstrual cycles. These are chemical messengers produced in one part of the body but active in another part. The control begins in the higher portions of the brain including the hypothalamus, which sends messengers (hormones) to the so-called master gland of the body (pituitary gland). This master gland, in response to the messages, makes its own hormones that travel to the ovaries. They stimulate the ovary to produce the egg cells and two hormones called estrogen and progesterone. It is the sudden fall in estrogen and progesterone production each month that leads to menstrual bleeding.

MENSTRUAL SYMPTOMS

Some of the menstrual symptoms are, of course, common to most women. Almost all experience some form of drawing and aching in the lower back and perhaps some abdominal cramps. The intensity and duration of these symptoms vary greatly from woman to woman and from month to month. Heightened emotional states seem to worsen them, too. Some women retain fluid just before their periods begin. They often feel bloated. Their ankles and feet swell. In addition to these familiar physical symptoms, some women also complain of fatigue, weakness, headaches, and even emotional ups and downs at the time of their periods.

MENOPAUSE

It is not surprising that most women have intense emotional reactions to any change in their menstrual cycle. The most dramatic change in the menstrual cycle is cessation of regular bleeding. When menstrual bleeding stops permanently, we say that the woman has reached menopause. This usually means no menstrual period has occurred for a year. Menopause rarely occurs before the age of forty, only 25 percent of the time before forty-five, and almost 100 percent of the time by age fifty-five.

This is a very significant time in your life. You suddenly realize that your childbearing years have ended, and you may have feelings of inadequacy and loss of vitality. You may feel as though part of you is gone, and so you begin to worry about aging. You may think that you have passed the zenith of your physical powers. Some women understandably take a very morbid view of the future at this time. In men there is no real counterpart to this life crisis.

If you tend to be pessimistic and have periods of depression before the menopausal years, you may be prone to depression when you reach menopause. In fact, many women who have always seemed stable, energetic, and spirited become depressed, moody, and short-tempered around the time of menopause. If this happens to you, remember you have lots of company.

You may find that you have great swings of mood at this time. You may be irritable, depressed, and hostile on one day and euphoric the next day. You may find also that you are more emotional and sensitive to happenings around you. You may have spontaneous crying spells or respond more profoundly and emotionally to a painting, concert, or play. In short, you may temporarily take on a new personality unrecognizable to yourself or your friends. Don't worry. You are having rough times, but they will pass.

Menopause does not usually come on suddenly. Generally, you will notice some gradual but significant changes in your menstrual cycles as you approach menopause. Sometimes, heavy, irregularly spaced menstrual periods signal the end of fertility. In most cases, this is followed by gradually scantier and less frequent periods for at least six months prior to the end of bleeding. Therefore, your psychological changes may start well before full menopause, and the relationship between the two may not be apparent to you or others. Once these menopausal psychological changes begin, they may last for several years. So it is very important to see their relationship to menopause. Unfortunately, middle-aged women may arouse the anger of family, friends, and business associates while going through menopause when they really need sympathy and understanding.

HOW TO COPE WITH THE CHANGES

What can you do to avoid or minimize these psychological effects of menopause? First of all, you need a realistic understanding of what menopause means. It is not a sign of generalized aging. It simply means that you are maturing. Cessation of menstrual flow does not mean that you have lost your vitality; you just cannot have a baby. That's all it means. You haven't lost your mental faculties or your ability to participate in physical exercise, or carry a normal workload, or enjoy sexual activity. In short, you are still the same person you were before you started having menopausal symptoms. Furthermore, there are definite advantages to reaching menopause. No longer do you have to worry about sanitary napkins to prevent messy bleeding, or about contraception to prevent unwanted pregnancy. You can live your life free of inconvenience, uncomfortable sensations, and sexual restraints. You can be a freer and more relaxed woman.

Secondly, recognize that your menopause has arrived and prepare yourself mentally. If you start to feel sorry for yourself, short-tempered, or lethargic, make a conscious effort to overcome these feelings. Refuse to give in. The best way to do this is to be actively involved in your family, friends, community, and hobbies. Choose a close friend in whom you can confide your personal feelings about what is happening to you. And don't forget your doctor. He can help you understand and cope with your new sensations and problems.

Most important, don't confuse the issue with other concerns. All women have a normal range of problems with their marriages, children, relatives, jobs, friends, companions, and with themselves. These are lifetime concerns. They won't go away, though, in time, they may become easier to bear and handle. The new and often unrecognized stresses of menopause tend to aggravate all the other problems. So, it's very important to keep these two sets of problems separate, and to try to deal with them separately. It's not easy. But you can do much to lessen the stresses of the menopausal period by learning to recognize their causes.

HOT FLASHES

The symptom most frequently associated with the menopause is "hot flashes." Many menopausal women complain of annoying and disconcerting episodes of flushing and hot sensations. These symptoms may occur frequently throughout the day (although not usually at night) and really have a wearing effect, resulting in fatigue and irritability. They are usually over in one to two years. No one really knows precisely what causes these hot flashes. However, the drop in circulating estrogen level seems to correlate best with the symptoms.

Fear seems to play a large role in aggravating the situation. Speak to your physician and let him reassure you. In most cases, reassurance about the absence of any disease makes it easier to cope with the symptom. It is interesting to note that 90 percent of women physicians have little or no trouble with hot flashes when they reach menopause.

ESTROGEN AND MENOPAUSE

What happens in the body to cause the process we have just described? Simply stated, menopause occurs when the ovaries run out of eggs. Follicles no longer develop and estrogen levels therefore become much lower.

One of the great controversies in today's medicine revolves around this question: Should women take estrogen pills after they reach menopause? There is no question that estrogen relieves some of the menopausal symptoms. It certainly seems to have a beneficial effect on the hot flashes, giving significant relief to some women who would otherwise be troubled by these wearing symptoms for months or even years. Most women, of course, pass through their menopause with only minor flashes that do not bother them much.

Estrogen has often been prescribed for depression and other personality changes even when there are no hot flashes. Here we believe the evidence is weaker. There is no evidence that depression is caused by hormone changes themselves and there is no reason to believe that estrogen will help. Depression must be dealt with through reassurance, counseling, and occasionally, antidepressant medications.

What about long-term estrogen use? Some doctors believe that it is worthwhile for postmenopausal women to take estrogen pills indefinitely. They feel that maintaining female hormone levels provides significant benefits for their patients and keeps them sexually youthful with a better self-image. In fact, if women take the pills for about twenty days and then stop for five days, some may have monthly bleeding, simulating their premenopausal state. There is no doubt that some women feel vital, more cheerful, and happier with this therapy. They can virtually ignore the fact that they have passed their fertile time of life. Why not then prescribe estrogen for all postmenopausal women?

Unfortunately, some women may pay a high price for their estrogen therapy. Like many medical therapies, estrogen therapy has serious side effects. These must be taken into consideration. Several important medical centers have collected statistics showing that postmenopausal women who take estrogen pills may get cancer of the uterus more often than women who are not on estrogen therapy. Uterine cancer is an extremely high price to pay for a better self-image.

There are other aspects to the estrogen debate. We know that fewer young women have hardening of the arteries and heart attacks than young men. After women reach the menopause and their estrogen levels go down, they start to catch up to men. Women who have their ovaries or even just their uterus removed at an early age are more likely to have heart attacks. It would seem logical, therefore, to assume that estrogen might provide some protection against hardening of the arteries especially in young women. The trouble with this theory, however, is that it runs counter to other observations. Women taking oral contraceptive pills (which contain estrogen) and men with prostatic cancer treated with estrogen actually have heart attacks more frequently. So at this time, the evidence about the effects of estrogen seems contradictory at best. The most recent evidence suggests that estrogen pills will not protect you against a heart attack.

Another potential advantage to taking estrogen has to do with your bones. We know that some women after menopause begin to lose calcium from their bones. This leads to softening of the bones (*osteoporosis*). Some experts have suggested that estrogen might prevent these changes, but this is also unproven.

Clearly, then, the decision for or against estrogen therapy is not an easy one. Your doctor must take many factors into account: how severe your symptoms are, how they are affecting your disposition, and your ability to deal with your problems.

If you are experiencing acute or disabling distress from flushing, we would choose estrogen treatment for a few months. Staying on this medication for a long time would, in our opinion, expose you to serious risks. Should you decide to undertake any estrogen treatment, you should do it knowing what the risks are. If you do take estrogen even for a short time, you should see your physician regularly. In our opinion, postmenopausal women should not take estrogen continuously for long periods of time.

PROBLEMS AFTER MENOPAUSE

Most postmenopausal problems are not particularly serious, but they can be quite distressing. For example, the lining of the vagina and skin around it depend on estrogen to keep it moist and healthy. Estrogen stimulates the lining cells to grow and certain specialized cells to produce lubricating liquid. After menopause, the lining may eventually become dry and thin. The dryness may lead to a bothersome vaginal itch. This itch can be treated by application of an estrogen cream.

With the loss of lubrication, the vagina becomes more susceptible to certain infections. Two parasites in particular often live in the vagina. One is a fungus called Monilia, and the other Trichomonas. Both of these microscopic creatures may produce a vaginal discharge and itching. The vaginal discharge, if profuse, may cause staining of underclothes. Monilia produces a thick, white, cheeselike fluid while Trichomonas' fluid is more watery, yellow, and thinner. Your family doctor or gynecologist can easily diagnose these conditions during a pelvic examination and prescribe effective treatment.

THE FALLING PELVIS

Another function of estrogen is to strengthen the ligaments and muscles that support the vault of the vagina, urethra, and urinary bladder. After estrogen levels have been low for a considerable period of time, these structures may begin to sag. Some women in their sixties and seventies, therefore, may be prone to prolapse of the bladder (*cystocele*) and uterus—so-called dropped womb. Women who have had many pregnancies may develop this problem even earlier.

When the uterus prolapses, it slips down in the vagina and may even protrude through the lips, especially with coughing. It is not painful but certainly quite disconcerting. In most cases, the degree of prolapse is minimal and requires

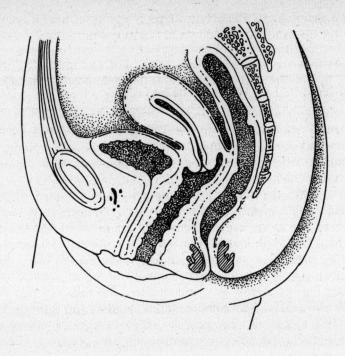

Fig. 25   Relationship of uterus, vagina, and bladder.

no treatment. With a moderate amount of prolapse, a plastic
or rubber support (pessary) can be inserted into the vagina
to support the uterus. This often holds the uterus in good
position. If the pessary or position of the uterus causes significant discomfort, it may be necessary in some cases to
perform pelvic surgery and remove or repair the uterus. This
is not a minor operation and should be avoided if possible in
older women.

   With changes in the position of the bladder, you may
find yourself urinating very frequently and without warning.
Characteristically, coughing or any sudden motion may
cause uncontrollable dribbling of urine because the bladder
sphincter is not in proper functioning position. This symptom is called *stress incontinence*. If you are seriously in-
convenienced by this problem, your physician can refer you

to a gynecologist for pelvic surgery. Again, although results of the operation are excellent, it is a major procedure.

ABNORMAL VAGINAL BLEEDING

A most important symptom in a woman of any age is abnormal vaginal bleeding. In a postmenopausal woman, of course, any vaginal bleeding is abnormal and requires prompt medical attention. In menstruating women, it is more difficult to know when the bleeding is abnormal. Certainly any bleeding between periods is abnormal as is the occurrence of menstrual periods at significantly shorter intervals. More difficult to notice but equally important is the onset of heavier periods: periods that last two to three days longer, require more sanitary napkins, or are associated with clots.

Unusual vaginal bleeding may result from a myriad of causes. It is always essential to rule out cancer of the uterus or cervix, especially in postmenopausal women in whom vaginal bleeding is very unusual. Your gynecologist will recommend a full examination including Pap smear, and then usually a uterine scraping (dilation and curettage). Under anesthesia, he will scrape the lining of the uterus so that it can be examined under the microscope. The results of the scraping will determine the best treatment for each woman.

CANCER

The chances of curing both cervical and uterine cancers are excellent if they are caught in the early stages. Depending on the situation, cervical cancer may be treated with radiation, surgery, or both, while cancer of the uterus always requires a total removal of the uterus. Even if the scraping does not show cancer, there may be evidence of a thickened uterine lining. This thickening, called *endometrial hyperplasia*, may predispose to cancer. It can sometimes be treated with hormones but may require a second scraping and sometimes a hysterectomy.

Fortunately, the scraping test usually rules out cancer, and so your gynecologist can turn his attention to any local, benign problem that may be causing bleeding. Sometimes the cause can be as simple as a benign polyp on the cervix, which can be seen on pelvic examination and easily removed.

FIBROIDS

The most common cause of increased bleeding in a menstruating woman is the presence of fibroid tumors of the uterus (*leiomyomas*). These are local areas of overgrowth of the muscle layer of the uterus that often can be felt on abdominal or pelvic examination. They are almost always benign and not dangerous unless they cause considerable bleeding. If there is enough bleeding to cause anemia, or if these fibroids become very large, bulky, and painful, it may be necessary to remove the uterus (hysterectomy). Fibroids tend to grow with estrogen stimulation and sometimes shrink after menopause. If the bleeding is only mild, it may make sense to be patient and perhaps avoid an operation. Secondly, the ovaries should not be removed during a hysterectomy for fibroids. Early loss of ovaries increases your chances of having heart attacks or weak bones (osteoporosis) later.

BREAST CANCER

It is estimated that 7 percent of all women born in the United States will have cancer of the breast at some point in their lives. The incidence of breast cancer rises with age and is most common in the postmenopausal decades, but a number of cases appear in young women. Unfortunately, we do not yet seem to be able to cut down the number of deaths from breast cancer. Breast cancer death rate has fallen only slightly in fifty years despite new diagnostic and therapeutic techniques for dealing with it.

We do, however, know a great deal more about breast cancer than we did a few years ago, and this information can be very helpful if properly applied. We know, for example, that certain women are at higher risk for contracting breast cancer than the general population. They include:

1. Women whose mothers had breast cancer
2. Women with multiple cysts in their breasts
3. Older women who have never had children.

We cannot prevent breast cancer because we do not know what causes it. But we can try to find it at an early stage when a cure is possible.

The first step is education. Every adult woman over thirty-five should be taught how to examine her own breasts for a lump. A doctor can show one how. She should do this regularly, at least once a month. In addition, she should know about two screening tests called *mammography* and *thermography*.

Mammography is an X-ray test that outlines a small mass in a breast that may be too small to feel with the fingers. Thermography is a highly sensitive procedure for measuring the skin temperature of each area of the breast. Cancer causes an increase in skin temperature.

It is not economically feasible to screen every woman regularly with these techniques. Furthermore, there is some concern that a woman who receives mammography annually may be exposed to too much radiation. All this radiation is probably not justified for most women. However, high-risk women should be considered for these procedures. If you are in a high-risk group, your physician may want you to have yearly mammography.

BREAST SURGERY

If you have a lump in your breast, the lump must be removed. If it is benign, nothing else is removed. If it is cancer, the surgeon will remove the breast (a *mastectomy*), and remove the lymph nodes under your arm on the same side. Surgery may be followed by a few weeks of radiation treatment to make sure that any remaining cancer cells are killed.

If the lymph nodes are found to have cancer in them, you may be referred to a specialist who will administer a course of anticancer drugs (*chemotherapy*). These drugs may temporarily weaken you and upset your stomach. You may have some nausea and vomiting, but these symptoms will pass. Some recent studies suggest that this treatment can be very effective and help cure you of the cancer.

HORMONE TREATMENT OF CANCER

The other treatment of breast cancer involves hormones. When a breast cancer is removed, a piece of it should be tested in the laboratory to see whether it combines with estrogen and progesterone (*receptor site test*). If it does, and if there is evidence that cancer has spread to other parts of the body, hormonal therapy is advisable. If you have breast cancer, make sure that your operation is performed in a hospital that can arrange for testing your cancer with estrogen and progesterone.

DEALING WITH LOSS OF A BREAST

It is not surprising that most women are depressed after losing a breast. After all, it is not pleasant to feel that a part of your femininity has been removed and that you have been a cancer victim. It will take time to get over this shock. But take heart because of what is available to you today. First of all, if your cancer is caught early and removed, your chances of being cured are excellent. Even if it was more advanced, you have a good chance of cure or at least controlling the cancer with chemotherapy or hormone treatment.

As for the loss of a breast, in no way should this permanently affect your vitality or sexuality. If you are concerned about the cosmetic appearance, you can use a mechanical prosthesis under your dress or even have it surgically implanted under the skin.

SUMMARY

There are a host of special medical problems that apply only to women, and most of them increase in frequency with aging!

1. The menopause is a dramatic time in a woman's life but should not be a cause for concern.

2. Psychological changes at the menopause are easier to handle if you realize that they will pass and if you can separate them from other aspects of your life.

3. Estrogen treatment for prolonged periods is dangerous, and estrogen must be used with extreme caution.

4. Unusual vaginal bleeding or postmenopausal bleeding is an important warning sign and indicates the need for a diagnostic scraping procedure.

5. Your uterus and ovaries should not be removed unless necessary. Before you have a hysterectomy for anything but cancer, discuss with your doctor what he plans and what you want. It may even be wise to ask for a second opinion. Remember that medicine is still an art, not an exact science.

6. Breast cancer can be dealt with effectively if diagnosed early. Every woman should learn how to examine her own breasts.

7. You should have a pelvic examination with Pap smear at least once a year.

13

GETTING UP WITHOUT GO: DIZZINESS AND WEAKNESS

As we grow older, we tire more easily. We can't do all the things we used to do. We can't do them as well or as long either.

Some people who keep fit by jogging or exercising or playing tennis regularly are able to maintain a fairly vigorous physical life well into their sixties and even seventies. But most of us, even though we enjoy good health in most other respects, commonly feel "tired," "weak," "listless," or complain of the "blahs."

Feeling tired or slowing up is part of the natural process of growing older, something to be expected and not to be alarmed about. But feeling weak or tired isn't always just a matter of getting older. These feelings are very often signals that something is wrong somewhere in the extraordinarily complicated mechanisms of your body. If you feel tired and weak, don't assume that there's nothing wrong with you simply because you are getting older. See your doctor and let him check you. There are a number of common conditions that cause weakness and tiredness.

ANEMIA

One of the most common causes of weakness and sluggishness is *anemia*. In anemia, there are not enough red blood cells in your blood. Your blood normally carries three kinds of cells, each with a different function. The *white blood cells* fight infection, the *platelets* prevent bleeding, and the *red blood cells* carry oxygen. It is the red blood cells that pick up oxygen in the lungs, carry it throughout the body, and give the oxygen to all the other cells of the body. Oxygen is carried inside the red blood cells by a substance known as *hemoglobin*.

If there are not enough red blood cells, the body does not receive sufficient oxygen and cannot utilize its fuel (food) for energy. Obviously anemia cuts down your energy and makes you feel tired. Someone with anemia may have dizzy spells, faint easily, complain of headaches or shortness of breath, and suffer from severe inertia. The anemic patient is like a heating system with a full fuel tank but no air to burn the fuel. He is, in a sense, suffering from a kind of low-grade asphyxiation. The anemic person takes oxygen into his lungs, but the oxygen does not get into his circulation. Without oxygen, no part of the body can function properly.

How badly one is affected by anemia depends not only on how serious it is, but also on how rapidly it develops. The human body has remarkable ways of compensating for many disorders, including anemia. If the number of red cells decreases very slowly over a period of months, symptoms may be very mild. The body learns to make use of the remaining red blood cells more efficiently so that they give up their oxygen to other cells more easily. On the other hand, if you have a severe bleeding episode and become anemic within a few hours or days, you may feel very weak, dizzy, and even faint.

If you come to your doctor feeling weak or tired, the first test he will order is a *blood count*, which will tell him how much hemoglobin and how many red blood cells you have. In fact, this test is always performed as part of an annual checkup, so that many people learn they have anemia before they have symptoms. Once your physician diagnoses anemia, his work has just begun. He must proceed in an orderly and logical fashion to try to find the cause of your anemia in order to treat it correctly.

After looking at your red blood cells under a microscope, your doctor will often want a *bone marrow test* performed. All three cells—white cells, red cells and platelets—are formed in the center (marrow) of the bones of the spine, skull, pelvic, breastbones, and part of the upper arm and thighbones. In order to find out more about your anemia, a blood doctor (hematologist) draws a small specimen of marrow through a needle inserted into the upper part of the breastbone (sternum) or pelvic bones.

IRON DEFICIENCY

Lack of iron in the blood is a very important cause of anemia. Iron is an essential part of hemoglobin (and is actually the material that holds and releases oxygen). Without iron, the bone marrow cannot make enough red blood cells and those that are made have little hemoglobin in them. The bone marrow test in an anemic person shows an absence of iron.

Growing children and pregnant women may lack iron because of dietary deficiency. Many young women are deficient in iron when they have heavy menstrual periods.

In postmenopausal women and in men of all ages, iron deficiency is a clue to abnormal bleeding somewhere in the body, most frequently in the gastrointestinal system. If you have iron deficiency, your physician will examine a specimen of stool for blood. Special X-ray tests, including an upper gastrointestinal series and barium enema, are needed to locate the cause of bleeding. If these tests do not reveal the cause of the bleeding, your doctor may want you to be examined with a colonoscope, an instrument that can be inserted into your colon through the rectum. Most abnormalities in the colon can be seen directly through this tube. This procedure is slightly uncomfortable, but very safe.

Older people may bleed from simple *hemorrhoids* (piles) or little *outpouchings* in the colon called *diverticulae*. Bleeding may be due to more serious ailments such as stomach *ulcers* and *cancer of the colon*. The best advice: At the first sighting of blood in the stool, see your doctor immediately. If you have cancer of the colon and discover it in its early stage, a surgical cure is still probable.

The standard treatment for iron-deficiency anemia is *iron pills*. If you take enough of these pills for several weeks, the anemia may improve no matter what the underlying cause. But you cannot assume that a good response to iron eliminates the need for further tests. Even if you feel very healthy, your physician must continue to look for the cause of your iron deficiency as quickly as possible.

VITAMIN DEFICIENCY

A second common cause of anemia is a deficiency of a vitamin called *folic acid*. Our bone marrows require small amounts of this vitamin to make red blood cells, and this is well supplied by a normal diet. However, people who have difficulty digesting their food, vomit a great deal, or have certain types of chronic diarrhea can become deficient in folic acid within a few months. Food faddists, alcoholics, and people deprived of fruits and vegetables may also not have enough folic acid. It is not uncommon, for example, for elderly people living alone on a very unbalanced diet to develop this kind of anemia. Small amounts of folic acid added to the diet will eliminate it.

An anemia very similar to folic-acid deficiency results from a lack of vitamin B_{12}. We become deficient in B_{12} only if we cannot absorb it from our intestines into the bloodstream. This can happen for two reasons. One reason relates to the functioning of the intestines themselves. Any disease that interferes with our ability to absorb food and vitamins into the bloodstream may cause B_{12} and/or folic-acid deficiency.

The other cause of B_{12} deficiency is known as *pernicious anemia*. In this disorder, the stomach fails to make a certain protein called *intrinsic* factor. Vitamin B_{12} cannot pass from the intestines to the bloodstream without the help of intrinsic factor, and so anemia gradually develops. The onset of pernicious anemia is very slow because the body usually has a lot of stored vitamin B_{12} in the liver that can tide it over for many months.

Vitamin B_{12} is needed by the brain, spinal cord, and nerves, as well as the bone marrow. Therefore, lack of vitamin B_{12} from any cause can lead to many neurological problems including weakness or paralysis of the legs, loss of sensation, and mental confusion. These neurological problems are more likely to arise if you receive only folic acid pills when you really have B_{12} deficiency. It is very important that your doctor determine whether you have folic acid or vitamin B_{12} deficiency. If he isn't sure which you have, he should treat you for both simultaneously or try vitamin B_{12} before he tries folic acid.

The treatment of vitamin B_{12} deficiency is a monthly injection of vitamin B_{12}. In pernicious anemia, you will have to take these injections all your life. Unfortunately, there are many physicians who give these injections for all sorts of conditions, including anxiety, change of life symptoms, and depression. This is just a waste of money. Vitamin B_{12} treatment is of value only for people with a real deficiency.

DRUG TOXICITY

Sometimes a medication prescribed for an entirely different illness produces anemia. Drugs used to treat arthritis, hyperactive thyroid gland, cancer, epilepsy, high blood pressure, infections, and many other conditions occasionally prevent the bone marrow from working properly. Fortunately, this rarely happens, but there is no way of predicting to whom it will happen. When this does occur, the white blood cells and platelets generally also suffer, so that infection or bleeding, rather than anemia, may be the first sign of trouble.

Most people with drug-induced anemia recover, but a few drugs are notoriously fatal. The worst offender is an antibiotic called chloramphenicol. This should never be prescribed except for a few infections that cannot be treated with any other antibiotics. It is really needed only for treating some kinds of meningitis and typhoid fever in people who are allergic to penicillin. Even then the patient must be carefully watched for signs of dangerous side effects.

DYING RED CELLS

The anemias that we have just discussed all have one thing in common. The bone marrow cannot manufacture enough red blood cells. Anemia can also occur with a normal bone marrow if the red blood cells do not live as long as they should. Normally each red blood cell lives for an average of one hundred and twenty-five days before being "buried" in the liver or spleen and replaced by a new one from the bone marrow. The iron from these dead cells is reclaimed and sent back to the bone marrow.

There are many diseases that shorten the life span of the red cells. If these cells die prematurely, even a hard-working bone marrow cannot keep up with the losses, and the individual becomes anemic. Skin and eyes often turn yellow because of the accumulation in the blood of a yellow pigment called bilirubin, which comes from broken-down hemoglobin. In older people, this kind of anemia is usually the result of a medication or a cancer of the lymph glands (lymphoma). To discover lymphoma requires extensive testing, but effective treatment is available in most cases.

THYROID PROBLEMS

Another fairly common cause of weakness and lethargy is an underactive thyroid gland (*hypothyroidism*). The thyroid is situated at the base of the neck just in front of the windpipe, where it produces a hormone called *thyroxine*. Thyroxine circulates throughout the body and has a profound effect on what happens in the body. For example, it controls our rate of metabolism and therefore determines how fast our cells can carry out their various jobs. Our appetite, weight, and general level of energy depend on our rate of metabolism. If our thyroid becomes sluggish, we become sluggish. The most prominent symptoms of an underactive thyroid (hypo-

thyroidism) are listlessness, weakness, lethargy, cold intolerance, and sometimes even mental confusion. People often
move, think, and speak slowly and quietly. Since these may
be the only symptoms of an underactive thyroid, doctors
routinely order a test to measure the amount of thyroxine in
the blood for anyone complaining of tiredness. Other signs
that may point to underactive thyroid include a slow pulse
rate, a coarse, low-pitched voice, puffiness of the face, loss of
the outer third of the eyebrows, cold intolerance, anemia,
and mild to moderate weight gain. The widespread impression that people with hypothyroidism are very much overweight is not true. Most people with underactive thyroid
glands are of normal or slightly above normal weight.

Thyroxine pills, taken daily and for the rest of your life,
will eliminate all the abnormalities caused by underactive
thyroid glands.

BLOOD ABNORMALITIES

There are chemical abnormalities in the blood that lead to
weakness and tiredness. We have already discussed low
blood-sugar levels and their effect on the body's functioning.
Lack of this fuel weakens muscles and damages the brain. In
addition to sugar, the concentration of other substances in
blood is critical to our functioning.

The most important of these substances are certain
minerals, including sodium and potassium. If the blood level
of either of these minerals is low, you may feel weak and
tired (and can even become paralyzed). With a low sodium
concentration, you may also become confused or emotionally upset. These abnormalities can be caused by vomiting,
diarrhea, kidney problems, or the injudicious use of water
pills (diuretics).

Kidney disease itself may cause weakness even if the
mineral levels are normal. When the kidneys fail to function
properly, many waste products such as urea cannot be eliminated from the body and accumulate in the blood. Early

symptoms are progressive weakness, lassitude, and insomnia. One clue to kidney failure is a change in sleeping pattern. People with failing kidneys often suffer from insomnia at night and sleep during the day. A simple blood test can quickly tell your physician whether your kidneys are functioning properly. (For full discussion of kidney problems, see chapter 11.)

INFECTION

There are many bodily infections that leave people feeling weak and "rotten" a good part of the time. Thirty years ago, tuberculosis rated high among these conditions. Largely because of less crowded living conditions, improved diet, better sanitation, early detection programs, and effective antibiotics, the prevalence of tuberculosis has dropped sharply in the United States in the last few decades. Only poor and overcrowded areas see many new cases today. Nevertheless, some middle-class, middle-aged, and older people still come down with tuberculosis.

Who may develop tuberculosis? To answer this question, we need to know something about the natural history of this infection. Tuberculosis is caused by bacteria (*tubercle bacilli*) that are very hardy and difficult to kill even with strong antibiotics. These bacteria can also lie dormant inside our white blood cells for many years (unlike most other bacteria that die after being swallowed by these cells). A sizable percentage of today's middle-aged and older people were brought up under conditions that exposed them to tuberculosis. Many of them actually contracted a form of tuberculosis at the time. But they showed no symptoms. A chest X-ray may reveal a small scar in the lungs or a skin test may be positive for tuberculosis. However, over the years these people did not suffer any ill effects from the tubercle bacilli in their bodies. Even after forty years or more, the right stress or combination of conditions can make these dormant bacteria active again. This stress can be a pregnancy relatively late in life, the development of diabetes, or some other serious disease, a period of poor nutrition, chronic diarrhea, or even overwork and insufficient sleep.

When tuberculosis "lights up," it usually causes lung infection with fever, night sweats, and coughing. The person may even cough up some blood. The tuberculosis may develop in other areas, such as the kidneys or bone marrow, and present puzzling symptoms. A case in point is that of Eleanor Roosevelt who had anemia, weight loss, and weakness and was thought to have cancer. Only after she died was it discovered that her bone marrow was loaded with tuberculosis. If you are feeling weak and losing weight, your doctor should check you for possible tuberculosis. This check requires a chest X-ray and a simple skin test. Fortunately, with our present array of antibiotics and other medications, tuberculosis can be cured in almost all people, if caught early enough.

INFECTIONS OF THE HEART

An infection of a heart valve (bacterial endocarditis) can also lead to slow, progressive weakness over a period of time. These valves are delicate structures that open and close in response to pressure built up by the pumping of the heart. They allow blood to come into the pumping chambers (ventricles) from the veins and to flow from these chambers into the arteries. In many people, these valves become scarred either by rheumatic fever or the wear and tear of years of opening and closing. These scarred valves are very susceptible to infection.

Even usually harmless bacteria in your throat, gastrointestinal system, and skin can invade these damaged valves. Infections of the valves are most likely to develop during some kind of operation. Thus, even a minor dental procedure may force some mouth bacteria into the bloodstream, allowing them to land on a damaged valve. So, before you undergo any surgical procedure, find out whether you have any heart valve abnormalities. Your physician can easily determine this by listening to your heart with a stethoscope. If he finds any abnormality, he will order an antibiotic for you on the day of your operation and for two days afterward.

If you develop a heart valve infection, you will have symptoms like anemia, heart murmur, low-grade fever, and sometimes little bleeding points on the skin or blood in the urine. Your physician can confirm this diagnosis by taking several blood specimens for "culture." The invading bacteria in the blood grow on special material (culture media) and can then be identified under the microscope. Treatment with antibiotics is very effective in curing this condition.

DIZZINESS

At one time or another, practically all of us become dizzy or faint. The experience is almost always pretty disturbing and frightening. Sometimes, this occurs because of anxiety, sudden fright, or news of an unexpected tragedy. This is understandable. But when dizziness or faintness occurs repeatedly and without an emotional trigger, you must seek medical advice. Dizziness, as we shall be using the term broadly here, is characterized by feelings of lightheadedness, loss of balance, and spinning sensations.

One of the most important and frequent causes of dizziness and fainting in middle-aged and elderly people is an abnormal heart rhythm (*arrhythmia*). This can develop in people with no history of heart disease and may be difficult to detect and diagnose. The electrocardiogram taken on a routine visit to the physician's office may be perfectly normal because these rhythm disturbances occur only once in a while.

Since your doctor cannot be with you every minute of the day, he must find another way to detect these rhythm changes in your heart. This has become feasible only in the last five years. A special monitoring apparatus, which is really a constantly recording portable electrocardiogram machine, is now available. It is so light that you can strap it to your chest and wear it for a day or two while performing your normal activities. This record of your heart's activity is submitted to a computer that surveys the data and detects any changes in your heart rhythm even if they last for only a few seconds. It is important for you to record any light-headedness or feelings of weakness that you have during this period and the exact times when they occur. Then your doctor can determine whether these symptoms resulted from any changes in rhythm on your recording.

These changes in heart rhythm cause dizziness because they decrease the amount of blood going to the brain. This happens because the heart is beating either too slowly or too quickly. It is vitally important to treat this rhythm problem because a prolonged attack can lead to a stroke and even death. If the heart beats too slowly, this condition can be corrected by an artificial pacemaker. Installing a pacemaker was once (ten years ago) a dangerous procedure. Thanks to our new technology, it has become an easy and highly successful technique that saves thousands of lives every year. Rapid heart rates can be treated with a number of drugs, such as Digitalis, quinidine, and procainamide. Your physician will choose the appropriate one for your condition. Some people require both a pacemaker and one of these medications.

DIZZINESS AND THE EAR

Ear problems, especially in the inner ear, can cause severe dizziness. Most people do not realize that their ears have more than a hearing function. They act as stabilizers that enable you to keep your balance when you walk or change position from sitting to standing. If the inner ears aren't functioning properly, you will experience severe dizziness with a spinning sensation (*vertigo*) when your head changes position. Motion sickness and seasickness, familiar examples of this problem, occur when changes in position are too abrupt for the inner ear to respond properly.

Anything that affects the ears—such as wax on the outside and infection on the inside—can lead to this kind of dizziness. The disorder called *Ménière's disease* (see page 289) can lead to attacks of severe dizziness. Very often, it takes the services of an ear specialist to help in spotting the cause of dizziness.

An unstable blood pressure is another frequent cause of dizziness. Normally, when you change from a lying or sitting position to the standing position, certain important reflexes occur very quickly so that your blood pressure does not fall. If these reflexes do not work properly, gravity forces down your blood pressure, less blood reaches your brain, and dizziness and/or fainting result. This condition is called *orthostatic hypotension.*

Unstable blood pressure is frequently caused by the treatment for high blood pressure. All the drugs given to lower the pressure can affect the blood pressure reflexes. Many people are particularly sensitive to one or more of these drugs, and so your physician should check your standing and lying blood pressure if he is treating you for *hypertension.* This same problem can be caused by nerve damage from a number of diseases such as diabetes. Usually you can avoid these symptoms by learning to rise slowly from the sitting or lying position and perhaps wearing elastic stockings or leotards.

Dizziness can also be caused by a blockage of the blood as it comes from the heart. The valve between the heart and the main artery (*aorta*) normally allows the blood to leave the heart and go to the rest of the body. If this valve becomes scarred, it will not open properly, and not enough blood will leave the heart. This condition called *aortic stenosis* can deprive the brain of blood it needs. The resulting dizziness is worse when you move or exercise. Your physician can make this diagnosis by hearing a heart murmur. Treatment may require heart surgery.

Finally, dizziness can be related to a problem in the brain itself. The lower part of the brain, called the *cerebellum*, is responsible for controlling equilibrium and balance and preventing dizziness. Any disease that affects the lower part of the brain can cause a problem in the cerebellum or its pathways. In elderly people, brain-related dizziness is usually due to clogging of arteries in the lower brain. If this clogging is in small arteries, the best that your doctor can do is to give you some medicines that offer partial relief. However, blockage of larger arteries may be amenable to surgery (see page 95).

BRAIN TUMORS

Your doctor must always make sure that the dizziness is not caused by a brain tumor rather than a blocked artery. To do this, he may have to order a brain scan or even a *CAT scan*. Both brain and CAT scans are painless procedures. For the first time, they make it possible to look into the body without actually "invading" it. For a brain scan, a radioactive isotope is injected into an arm vein and a scanning machine is placed near the head. A tumor, if present, will react to this isotope, and the scanner will record a "hot spot" in the brain. A CAT scan is a new technique by which a whole set of X-rays of the head is taken simultaneously and analyzed by a computer. It gives a picture of the entire brain and makes it easy to pick out a tumor.

The most common brain tumor to cause dizziness is called an *acoustic neuroma*. It sits right on the nerve going to the ear and also causes hearing loss and ringing in the ears. Surgery for this tumor is very effective.

SUMMARY

Chronic weakness and tiredness or dizziness may be a signal of some malfunction deep within the body. How do you know when to be concerned about this symptom? A good rule of thumb is to go to your doctor if you find yourself weaker or more tired for more than a week, and do not know why.

14

ARTHRITIS
AND SORE JOINTS

There's a bottle of aspirin in everybody's medicine cabinet. But did you ever notice on those TV commercials who always seems to need aspirin? An older person, of course! As the commercial says, "... to combat the pains and misery of arthritis." The implication is clear: Only older people worry about arthritis. Nothing could be further from the truth! Some of the most crippling forms of arthritis frequently strike younger people. That is not to say that older people don't have their share of achiness and sore joints. But while these may cause some inconvenience they certainly don't produce the permanently pained expressions and exaggerated infirmity seen on the TV characters.

People often ask whether arthritis is the same as "rheumatism." Arthritis is a very specific condition, inflammation of a joint. "Rheumatism" is not a precise term. It enjoys wide popularity because it is a convenient way to indicate any

ache in a muscle or joint without requiring a definite diagnosis.

OSTEOARTHRITIS

If you notice more aches and discomfort in your joints with
each passing year, chances are that you have osteoarthritis.
For most people, this should not be a matter of concern. In
fact, even though it's called arthritis, it is in a large part the
natural consequence of the use, and sometimes abuse, of our
joints. For this reason, specialists prefer to use the term
"degenerative joint disease" when discussing this type of
joint problem. It's their way of saying that our joints are
showing signs of wear. To be sure, there is some pain, but
usually it is just a simmering, vague discomfort. However,
on occasion it may boil over into a more severe attack.

A joint should be looked upon as a hinge between two
bones. Although more complex, it is subject nevertheless to
the same type of swinging stresses. Not surprisingly, the friction caused by years of use eventually affects our joints. It
is remarkable how well they withstand this unending stress.
No iron hinge, no matter how sturdy, would wear as well.
Inevitably, some signs of wear will appear in all of us, but
most of us will scarcely be aware of it.

Some people are more distressed by the appearance of
their joints than by pain and physical limitation. But gnarled
fingers or enlarged joints rarely interfere with our movement
and are never as conspicuous as self-conscious people think
they are. What really lies just beneath the surface of most
people's complaints is the fear that the joint problem may
turn into a disabling condition. But they can rest easy.
Osteoarthritis will not lead to serious disability in most people.

In fact, many older people are surprised to learn that
their X-rays show signs of osteoarthritis. Their joints don't
bother them, they say. This is not unusual. The X-ray will
often show changes, sometimes quite marked, despite minor
or no pain.

WHICH JOINTS DEVELOP OSTEOARTHRITIS?

Some joints fare worse than others. Understandably, those joints that must support the heaviest load or which must meet constant demands are likely to be the first to show signs of wear. This is why our hips and the joints of our legs give us the most trouble. If there are days when your shoulder or knees move like the ratchet of a spring-wound clock, just remember how well they have served you over the years, and it shouldn't surprise you that they're somewhat worn now. Simple, normal, everyday activity is sufficient to cause osteoarthritis, although other unknown factors that we do not completely understand obviously play a role.

TREATMENT OF OSTEOARTHRITIS

You are going to be disappointed if you expect us to recommend the latest medicine with some unpronounceable name. Nothing has come along that's better overall than aspirin! For once, all those commercials are accurate. It is true that in recent years a number of aspirinlike substitutes (called *non-steroidal anti-inflammatory drugs*) have become available such as ibuprofen, naproxen or sulindac. All of these require a doctor's prescription. In individual cases, they may be more effective and even safer than aspirin, but many people still find that aspirin works the best for them.

Although it is a surprisingly safe drug, aspirin is not without its problems. The most serious one, internal bleeding, has received a great deal of publicity, particularly by manufacturers of aspirin substitutes. While the problem shouldn't be minimized, aspirin is safe for most people if used properly.

1. Use only enough to reduce your discomfort.

2. Never take aspirin on an empty stomach! Try to take it with meals or, if not possible, with a good dose of liquid antacid.

3. Above all, never use aspirin as a sleeping pill. Avoid taking it at bedtime. But if you must use it for the nighttime pain, take liberal doses of antacid with it.

4. Anyone with an ulcer or, for that matter, with significant heartburn or stomach distress, should keep away from all forms of aspirin whether buffered or in effervescent tablets. An aspirin substitute that is readily available without prescription is acetaminophen (Tylenol, Datril). While it does not cause internal bleeding, it is often less effective for the nagging discomfort of osteoarthritis.

OTHER MEASURES FOR OSTEOARTHRITIS

Besides the judicious use of aspirin, there are other rules to follow that can help a person afflicted with osteoarthritis:

1. It is seldom necessary to take strong pain relievers for the treatment of osteoarthritis. But for those times when the joint throbs with changes in the weather, there are a number of medications your doctor can prescribe to make you more comfortable.

2. Cut down on physical activity when your symptoms flare up. This does not mean that you should not move around at all. On the contrary, you should exercise to maintain tone in the muscles around the joint. Simple common sense will tell you how much you can tolerate. Don't overdo it. Slow, gentle movement is enough.

3. Warm, moist heat is often quite helpful in relieving spasm and reducing the sensation of stiffening in the joint. A warm bath or shower serves the purpose particularly well when several joints are involved. Yet there are people who experience more discomfort when warmth is applied to the aching joint. Obviously, if this occurs in your case, it should be discontinued. Moist packs at room temperature may prove more suitable.

4. Reduce your weight if you are overweight. This will lessen the burden on weight-bearing joints, particularly hips, knees, and ankles, and in conjunction with other measures, help ease much of the daily discomfort.

SURGERY FOR OSTEOARTHRITIS

In a small number of people, irreparable damage to the joint can lead to severe distress and limitation of movement. This is not a sudden event. It develops over a period of years. It may progress so slowly that the individual is barely aware that his pace has slackened until he eventually moves with painful, measured steps. Thanks to dramatic advances in orthopedic surgery, it is now possible for many of these people to regain a good deal of their mobility. The most immediate benefits can be seen in people with serious hip problems. Although progress is being made in surgical treatment of most other joints, particularly the knee, elbow and wrist, the results have not equaled those of replaced hip joints. Even people with badly damaged hip joints can benefit from this procedure. It is remarkable how a shattered and frozen joint can be restored to a near full range of motion, and how doors are opened to a wide new world to people long confined to the narrow limits of their room or neighborhood.

Of course surgery is not for everyone, and not everyone will have the same results. The decision to undergo this operation must be made in full cooperation with your doctor. This remains a formidable surgical procedure despite refinement in skills and techniques. It may be too strenuous for people with serious heart, lung, or kidney ailments. Occasional infection of the artificial joint remains one of the more disturbing complications of the procedure, and will probably discourage the surgeon from recommending it in someone who already has serious infections elsewhere. But for a large number of patients the potential benefits far outweigh the risks.

GOUT

The person with gout must often feel doubly afflicted. Not only does he suffer the most acute pain in his swollen joints, but he's more likely to elicit amusement rather than sympathy from his friends.

Gout has been recognized for several thousand years, but few people will get any comfort out of knowing that they share a common misfortune with some of history's most notable figures. For centuries, cartoonists have delighted in caricaturing the gouty patients—everyone is familiar with a stereotyped figure sitting with his leg propped up, an immensely swollen toe peering from beneath rolls of bandages. But there's nothing funny about gout. It is a very, very painful condition. In our hapless cartoon figure, only the swollen toe is accurately represented since this joint is probably more frequently involved than any other. However, virtually any joint in the body can be afflicted, such as knees, ankles, wrists. While men seem to be unfairly singled out early in life, later in life both men and women are at equal risk. Gout seems to run in families.

CAUSE OF GOUT

In most types of arthritis, we do not know why the joints become inflamed. This is not the case with gout. Here, the culprit is a substance called *uric acid*, which forms deposits in the joints and causes the inflammation. Normally, this substance circulates freely in the bloodstream. Uric acid is formed in the body from compounds called *purines*, which are constituents of every body cell. It enters the bloodstream as part of the debris from the breakdown of remnants of worn cells in the body and is eliminated through the kidneys in the urine. In the gouty patient, an excessive amount of uric acid builds up in the bloodstream. For reasons which we still do not understand, the uric acid settles out as crystals in the joint. The effect of these crystals in the joint can be as explosive as a match touched to gasoline, igniting it into a painful swelling. In gout's worst form, the joints seem to be baking on a living hearth. Not all attacks are this severe. In many cases, the pain seems to be just smouldering over a low flame. Usually the pain erupts quite abruptly without much warning, although some people experience a more prolonged period of achiness. The attacks usually subside in a few days if untreated, and in a few hours if treated correctly. Between attacks, there are usually no symptoms. If left untreated, long-standing gout can be accompanied by the slow nibbling away of the joint and permanent injury. In some people, small lumpy deposits, called *tophi*, accumulate beneath the skin, often on the forearms or ears, but occasionally elsewhere. These lumps represent stony deposits of uric acid crystals that precipitate relentlessly from body fluids like stalactites condensing in a moist cave. Since they cause no pain, they can be easily overlooked until called to one's attention. Before modern methods of treatment, some of these deposits reached disfiguring sizes. Modern therapy has virtually eliminated these more destructive and disabling forms of gout.

Another consequence of elevated uric acid in the bloodstream is a tendency to form kidney stones. This disposition has probably been exaggerated in the past but those people who pass a large amount of uric acid in their urine seem to be at greatest risk. The urine may be unable to dissolve large amounts and the excess may precipitate out as stones. This is why people with gout are cautioned to drink large amounts of liquids. Newer drugs have eliminated much of the problem of kidney stones, however.

DIAGNOSIS AND TREATMENT OF GOUT

If a hot, swollen joint can be caused by a number of conditions, how can your doctor be sure that you are suffering from gout? Most of the time, the typical onset of the attack and the appearance of the joint together with a high level of uric acid in the blood is all that he needs to make a diagnosis of gout. To be absolutely certain, however, it is necessary to remove a very small amount of fluid from the joint and examine it under the microscope. The unmistakable presence of urate crystals in the fluid leaves no doubt that this is an attack of gout. Doctors often rely on inspection of the joint fluid to assist them in determining a precise cause of arthritis. At times, this affords only minor leads while in some instances the information may be crucial in determining how to treat the attack. A good example is the case of arthritis due to an infection of the joint. This type of arthritis requires prompt, specific treatment yet may look exactly like gout.

The successful treatment of gout is one of the triumphs of modern medicine. Not only can the misery of the acute attack be effectively doused but it is possible to reduce and often eliminate subsequent attacks. Different types of medicines are now available for these purposes. The sudden flareup requires a medication to combat inflammation. Phenylbutazone or indomethacin are very effective for this purpose. Both these drugs can be harsh on the intestinal tract and should be avoided by people with ulcers. Phenylbutazone must be used with caution by people with heart failure. Colchicine is an entirely different kind of medication that has been used successfully in the treatment of gout for centuries. How it acts is not precisely clear, but its ability to arrest a sudden attack of gout seems unique. In fact, this seems to be one of the few uses for this drug. So specific and dramatic is the response in gout that some doctors use it to make a diagnosis of gout. Some physicians prefer to inject it into a vein because the large number of tablets required for an acute flare-up can lead to severe diarrhea. After the flareup subsides it may be necessary to take one or two tablets per day for a while, but this dose seldom causes any problem.

One word of caution: Aspirin should never be used for the pain of gout. In doses that are ordinarily used, it can raise uric acid levels and actually cause an attack of gout.

After the acute attack subsides, your doctor will want you to take measures to prevent future attacks. There are several types of drugs available for this purpose. The one most commonly prescribed is allopurinol, which prevents the body from manufacturing uric acid from purines. While this drug is very effective, some people are unable to tolerate it because it has certain side effects, such as skin rash.

These people can substitute other types of drugs that lower uric acid levels by speeding its disposal through the kidneys. Because this increases the concentration of uric acid in the urine, this type of drug is not suitable for people with kidney stones. The most widely used drugs of this sort are probenicid and sulfinpyrazone. The latter drug has aroused recent excitement because of the preliminary evidence that it reduces death rate for at least six months following a heart attack. This makes it an ideal drug to use in patients with gout who have had a recent heart attack.

Gout is a lifelong problem. To prevent an attack, medicines must be taken indefinitely. If an attack occurs rarely, some doctors prefer to simply treat the acute attack rather than keep a person on medications permanently. This makes sense for the attack occurring every one or two years, but the patient experiencing frequent attacks would be better off with preventive medicines.

SOME TIPS FOR THE GOUTY PATIENT

If you have gout here are a few things you can do to help yourself:

1. Eat a regular, well-balanced diet. Don't skip meals and don't eat too much at one sitting. With medications it is no longer necessary to adhere to a rigid *purine-free* diet, although foods very high in these compounds should be avoided. Such foods as sweetbreads or red meats are high in purine content. Although it is the breakdown of purines that leads to the accumulation of uric acid in the body, most purines are actually made by your own body.

2. Avoid undue stress. Overexertion or trauma to a joint can lead to a gouty attack.

3. Get an adequate amount of sleep. Rest when you feel tired.

4. Keep warm in the winter. Don't forget the gloves and warm undergarments on chilly days.

5. Know your medicines. Some medicines can cause a gouty attack. We have already mentioned aspirin, but most water pills can do the same. Don't borrow pills from friends or use any medication without consulting your doctor. If you must use water pills for your heart or your blood pressure, your doctor can prescribe allopurinol along with them.

6. Remember to drink lots of fluid.

PSEUDOGOUT

The name "pseudogout" literally means "false gout." It is aptly named for it closely resembles gout and can be just as painful. In addition, crystals will be found deposited in the joint, although in this case they are calcium pyrophosphate rather than uric acid crystals. Unlike gout, there is no buildup of uric acid in the blood in pseudogout, and the dramatic response to medication so typical of gout is lacking. The onset of an attack can be as explosive as gout and, untreated, can last more than a week. The knees are most likely to be involved, but other joints can also be affected. If the attack is not too severe, an anti-inflammatory drug such as phenylbutazone is sufficient to bring relief. In some cases, removal of fluid from a badly swollen joint may be necessary. Some doctors inject cortisone into the joint at the same time if the situation warrants.

RHEUMATOID ARTHRITIS

Rheumatoid arthritis is the most destructive form of joint inflammation. Even though it most frequently strikes during the early years of life, its full consequences continue to be felt throughout life. While the most painful phase of the disease will have spent itself later in life, it leaves damaged joints in its wake. Sometimes an older person will develop rheumatoid arthritis for the first time.

In many ways, rheumatoid arthritis presents the greatest challenge of all joint disease to patient and doctor alike. As it advances, it spares no joint in the body, although knees, wrists, and hands seem to be particularly hard hit. In the long run, most people suffer only discomfort in the affected joints without any major disability. Yet we more often hear of the smaller number left with badly damaged joints. Rheumatoid arthritis remains a complex and poorly understood condition, often weakening the whole body as much as the joints.

TREATMENT OF RHEUMATOID ARTHRITIS

It is well beyond the scope of this book to go into any great detail about this many-sided condition. A good general rule followed by most physicians is to use the mildest effective medicines possible. Aspirin meets this objective best, especially when used in very high doses. A number of newer drugs, in some ways much like aspirin, have allowed doctors more variety in the type of medications they can prescribe. These include ibuprofen, naproxen, indomethacin, and tolmetin among others.

In the past, cortisone was widely used in treating rheumatoid arthritis. Today doctors are reluctant to use cortisone drugs for a condition that extends over many years. This is not to say that cortisone is not effective. It is, and usually dramatically so. But long-term use can thin bones, collapse the spine, and cause a number of other unpleasant side effects. While the arthritis pain may be well controlled, cortisone does nothing to halt the progressive destruction of the joint. Therefore most doctors try to avoid use of these drugs altogether or use them for short periods when the attack is most severe and then discontinue them as soon as possible. In those people who seem unable to exist without experiencing intolerable pain, the lowest possible dose should be used. Even then, every attempt should be made to switch to other types of medication.

Gold injections have enjoyed fluctuating popularity over the years. No one questions their effectiveness. They relieve symptoms in a good number of patients but require frequent injections, and take months before any results are noticed, too long for some people accustomed to the instantaneous results produced by other medications. In addition, they can lead to serious side effects, which must be closely watched for with blood and urine tests. For these reasons, doctors are reluctant to use gold injections in people with milder forms of rheumatoid arthritis. Nevertheless, they remain one of the most valuable forms of treatment for rheumatoid arthritis, providing lasting benefit for many people.

Chloroquin, a drug used to treat malaria, is occasionally used by some physicians. Because it can result in serious eye damage and requires frequent eye checkups, it is less often prescribed today.

Recently, a new drug called *penicillamine* has been introduced for the treatment of rheumatoid arthritis. Because it has many severe side reactions this drug is reserved for people with severe symptoms who fail to benefit from other medicines. The decision to use this medication must carefully weigh the potential benefit against potential harm.

PHYSICAL THERAPY

The most important strides in the treatment of rheumatoid arthritis have come with the recognition of the crucial role of exercise, physiotherapy, and splinting of joints to prevent crippling deformities. The entire physical therapy program requires close collaboration between physician and patient. The repetitive exercises often seem deceptively simple and monotonous, and it is easy to become frustrated if you expect immediate or dramatic results. Yet just such a program has made it possible to prevent some of the disabling deformities that restrict the life of the rheumatoid patient.

The basic principle of physiotherapy is simple enough: Exercise prevents deterioration of the muscles and stiffening of the joint. Thus, patients with rheumatoid arthritis should constantly remind themselves to move their joints and avoid remaining in one position for long periods. Special splinting devices may be necessary for some people, especially during sleep when fixed and abnormal positioning of the joint are likely to occur. Not everyone has need for such devices, however.

Of course, no amount of medicine or physical therapy can repair a joint badly deteriorated after years of inflammation. But thanks to exciting advances in orthopedic surgery, even people with the most disabling forms of arthritis have reason for hope. Function has been restored to even the most damaged joint, welded stiff from inflammation, by replacing it with an artificial one. This is now possible with hip, knee, and even elbow joints. Many people unable to walk or use their limbs have regained useful life through modern surgery. Of course, surgery has its limitations. Not everyone benefits to the same degree. In some people, surgery may not even be possible. However, with the collaboration of the orthopedist and experts in joint diseases, it is possible to decide beforehand just how much surgery has to offer in each individual case.

POLYMYALGIA RHEUMATICA

Sometimes the name of a condition is more fearsome than the disease itself. A good example is polymyalgia rheumatica. It's medical shorthand for "pains in many muscles and joints." The symptoms are extremely vague—persistent fatigue, weakness, cramplike muscle aches, and severe stiffness. With an almost perverse patience, this ailment waits for old age before it appears. It shouldn't be too surprising that with symptoms such as these, an older person has difficulty in finding someone who will take his complaints seriously. Generally, he's either ignored or treated with a condescending assurance that the aches will disappear if only he stops thinking too much about himself. It doesn't take too long to become frustrated or even to doubt if the symptoms are real.

To compound the difficulty there is no precise test to diagnose the condition. A simple test, called a *sedimentation rate*, is always abnormal in polymyalgia rheumatica, but it is also abnormal in many other conditions, including simple viral illnesses. Nevertheless, a persistently elevated sedimentation rate is a clue to the presence of polymyalgia. If you are over the age of sixty and have these vague symptoms, your doctor will probably ask for a sedimentation rate. If symptoms persist and he finds no other reason for the elevated sedimentation rate, he can make the diagnosis of polymyalgia rheumatica. Treatment with cortisone for a few months cures the condition.

While polymyalgia rheumatica itself is generally harmless, another condition called *temporal arteritis* occasionally accompanies it. This condition is an inflammation of arteries and often involves the arteries on the scalp. It may also involve arteries supplying blood to the brain and result in serious consequences, particularly sudden and often irreversible blindness. It is important therefore to exclude this latter condition in patients with polymyalgia rheumatica. A diagnosis is easily made by sampling a small piece of a blood vessel from the scalp and examining it under the microscope. If signs of inflammation are found, prompt treatment with cortisone will prevent the development of any eye problems. Treatment for at least a year is necessary.

ALL THAT ACHES IS NOT ARTHRITIS

Remember this the next time you feel a pain or ache in or around a joint. The first thing most people think of when this happens is that it must be arthritis. Most aches, however, are not caused by arthritis, but by inflammation or stretching of the structures surrounding the joint. Each joint is embraced by tough bindings called *ligaments* and straddled by powerful muscles with their fastenings called *tendons*. Deep-seated achiness and stiffness often arise from problems within these structures. A sprain, for example, is an over-stretching or tear in the ligaments tautly wrapped around the joints. *Fibrositis* is a term used by specialists to indicate an ill-defined, deep soreness and stiffness within the muscle abutting certain joints, although the exact source of the pain is unclear. For most of these conditions we have just talked about, warm, moist heat, gentle exercise with proper rest, and mild pain relievers like phenybutazone are all that is required. Sometimes an injection of a painkiller or cortisone into the area helps but this is generally reserved for severe pain.

Every now and then an inflammation of another structure can masquerade as arthritis and lead to some confusion. A case in point is *bursitis*. This is a swelling of a small fluid-filled sac, which covers the joint and acts normally as a ball bearing for the structures sliding over the joint (see Fig. 26). When it is swollen and tender, it may be difficult to distinguish it from arthritis. Mild inflammation of the bursa can also cause severe soreness, stiffness, and limitation of movement. An anti-inflammatory drug such as aspirin or

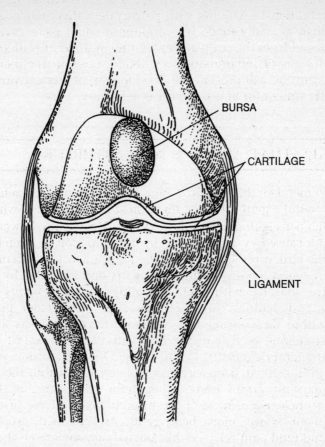

BURSA

CARTILAGE

LIGAMENT

Fig. 26   Knee joint. The thigh bone (femur) and the shin bone (tibia) are connected at the knee joint. A layer of softer material called cartilage lines two adjoining surfaces. The knee cap (patella) is a separate bone not shown here.

phenylbutazone will usually relieve the bursitis. If it is nagging and persistent, however, your doctor may suggest a cortisone injection into the affected bursa.

Unfortunately, on rare occasions more serious conditions can mimic arthritis. Irritation of nerves in the spine by a ruptured disc (see page 238) or tumor can cause pain resembling arthritis, often even pinpointed to one joint.

The point we want to make here is simply that many conditions may resemble arthritis yet have nothing to do with the joints. So don't jump to conclusions. Let your doctor make the diagnosis.

SUMMARY

1. Most pains and aches in joints are due to longtime wear and are rarely anything to be concerned about.

2. For people with the most serious forms of injury, newer surgical operations have restored excellent joint function, particularly in the hips.

3. Help in the form of newer drugs and better approaches to physical therapy have become available for many forms of arthritis.

4. A simple rule holds for any form of arthritis: Rest the joint when it is severely inflamed and begin simple exercises as soon as pain decreases.

15

BRITTLE BONES
AND ACHING BACK

To most of us a skeleton appears to be nothing more than a simple arrangement of uncomplicated parts geometrically well organized to support our body. But is it really that simple? Hardly! Rather than cold and lifeless girders, our bones are living tissue. When shattered, broken, or injured, they heal intact again, and our skeleton grows from infancy to adulthood. Drab and unglamorous though it appears, the bare skeleton is in every way as complex and as adaptable as any other part of our body. As we grow older, many changes occur in bone as elsewhere in our bodies. To understand why and how these changes take place, we need to know how normal bone behaves.

The sinister, dangling skeleton you've seen in laboratories is no more the normal skeleton than the molted shell is the living shellfish. For bone is a complex tissue composed of the chiseled, stony form we can see, superbly crafted by living cells that dwell within it, and cannot be seen with the naked eye. Although we cannot see it, bone is in a constant state of renewal. For deep within the bone, the living cells ceaselessly weave an exquisite lattice with the precision of the spider spinning its web. This lattice forms the scaffold upon which the bony structure is built up, like a cement superstructure poured upon a steel framework. Yet as a dynamic vital system, the whole structure is forever changing, as cells remove and rebuild the inner structure of bone like artists working with living clay.

OSTEOPOROSIS

Bones lose some of their compactness and some of their strength as we grow older. In this condition, known as osteoporosis, the fine mesh upon which bone is built loses its tightly knit arrangement and the entire bone becomes more spongy. For, like a woven fabric, the strength of bone depends upon its inner, woven mesh. Women are more prone than men to this gradual thinning of their bones and are more apt to develop problems from it.

The exact reason for these changes in the aging bone remains unclear. The decline of certain female hormones (see page 231) at the time of menopause may predispose women to the thinning of their bones. Perhaps because of male hormones, men seem to be less affected as they grow older. Another factor may be the requirement of bone for calcium to form its hard, cement structure. The diet of many people is deficient in calcium throughout their adult lives perhaps because they consume smaller quantities of milk and milk products than they did as children. A certain amount of calcium in the diet is required to produce bone of normal strength. If the body does not get the calcium it needs, the bones will eventually weaken. Just like muscle, bones require a certain degree of activity to keep up their tone and resilience. A tendency to do less physical activity may contribute to the thinning of bones in older people.

Few people notice that their bones have grown less sturdy. To a greater or lesser degree, all of us will develop some bone changes as we grow older. So subtle are these changes that even an X-ray examination may not detect them. Why be concerned at all about osteoporosis? Because in individual cases the less dense bone becomes too fragile, incapable of resisting undue stress. This is most likely to occur in the vertebrae, the building blocks of the spine, which can collapse if sufficiently weakened. You may have noticed that you are shrinking in height with the passing years. If you have lost an inch, it could be the result of collapse or shrinkage of your vertebrae. Surprising as it may seem, there may not be any pain when this happens. Some bones may unexpectedly fracture with a minor injury or fall.

One of the more disturbing examples of this phenomenon is the frequent occurrence of hip fractures in older people, following a seemingly insignificant fall or injury. This is all the more regrettable since many of these accidents are preventible, such as a fall from a stool while reaching towards a shelf or even missing the curb while walking. While women seem more likely to develop collapse of the vertebrae, both men and women are prone to hip fractures.

AVOIDING PROBLEMS WITH OSTEOPOROSIS

What can be done for osteoporosis? Once the bone has substantially weakened, there is not much that can be done to rebuild it. Still, it is the fractures resulting from the weakened bones that cause the real problems and in many cases you can do something about this. Be on guard at all times for situations that invite accidents. Here are a few examples of what you can avoid:

1. Your spine is pretty strong, but not strong enough to support any weight you choose to handle. So don't lift heavy packages. Get someone with a younger and sturdier spine to move those pieces of furniture, carry your heavy luggage, or shovel the snow.

2. Going for walks on icy days may be invigorating or a way to test if you're still as surefooted as you once were. But it's dangerous. Always stay on cleared pavement. Walk slowly and watch your footing.

3. Step carefully in and out of the bathtub or shower. Make sure there are readily accessible means to steady your balance, such as hand bars and a good dry nonslip mat or towel. It's also a good idea to place nonskid mats in the tub and shower.

4. Don't climb on chairs or makeshift ladders to reach a high shelf. Keep items that are used frequently within easy reach.

5. Beware of slippery waxed floors or loose carpets. They may seem innocent enough, but you're flirting with catastrophe each time you step on them.

6. Watch your footing while stepping down or up curbs. Cross at a light and give yourself enough time to cross without rushing.

7. Always use handrails while walking a stairway to keep a steady footing.

8. Take your time getting in and out of cars or buses. A few moments' wait should make no difference to the driver or other passengers.

This is obviously not a complete list, but there are enough suggestions here to alert you to what you should do to protect yourself against injury.

PREVENTION OF OSTEOPOROSIS

Of course it would be a lot more practical to prevent osteoporosis than to expend so much effort in avoiding actual and potential risks. Unfortunately, in most cases, we do not yet know enough about osteoporosis to be able to accomplish this. In certain cases we may find a definite, treatable cause, such as an overactive parathyroid gland, which causes loss of calcium in the urine. People on long-term cortisone drugs are particularly susceptible to this type of bone injury. This is one of the reasons why doctors continually try to reduce the dosage of cortisone drugs in people who must use them. In certain rare intestinal disorders, calcium and vitamin D may be poorly absorbed. The presence of persistent diarrhea or frequent bulky stools along with weight loss may be a clue to such disorders.

We need to know much more about the nature of bone thinning. But as of now the wise thing to do is to maintain a reasonable level of calcium in your diet. Three glasses of milk per day will meet normal daily requirements for calcium. Skim milk is just as rich in calcium as whole milk.

Other valuable sources of calcium include cheeses, green leafy vegetables such as spinach, and canned fish, such as sardines. Most milk is fortified with vitamin D, which is also essential for maintaining adequate calcium in the body. Cod liver oil provides sufficient amounts to meet body needs for this vitamin without risking taking too much. Ask your doctor if it would benefit you.

For those people who cannot get their daily calcium requirements into their diet, calcium tablets are available in pharmacies and food stores. One word of caution, however. Too much calcium can be just as harmful as too little. The amount of calcium in a normal diet or even that provided by recommended amounts of calcium tablets will not lead to excessive intake of calcium. However, vitamin D taken in too large quantities can lead to serious accumulation of calcium in the blood. So, before deciding to take any of these on your own, talk to your doctor.

A diet high in protein may cause the body to lose calcium. It seems reasonable, therefore, that people with significant osteoporosis should cut down the amount of protein in their diet. This is easily accomplished by switching from a high meat diet to a more balanced diet of vegetables and fruits. Certainly try to keep active. A brisk daily walk is invigorating and should keep your muscles and bones in tone.

Some authorities believe that fluorides may play a role in strengthening bones. While it does seem to be helpful, get some expert advice before deciding on this type of treatment.

FEMALE HORMONES AND OSTEOPOROSIS

For many years, we have known that older women are more likely than older men to develop osteoporosis. As we have mentioned previously (see page 228), the decline of female hormones at the time of menopause may in part be responsible. It seemed logical, therefore, to try to halt this process by replacing one of these hormones, *estrogen*. However, long-term treatment with this hormone still leaves doubt about its effectiveness. Of more immediate concern, however, is the unexpected number of women developing cancer of the uterus after many years on this medication. Widespread enthusiasm greeted this form of therapy at first. Today, that enthusiasm has waned considerably. Because of the dangers associated with the use of estrogen, most doctors do not treat osteoporosis this way today unless the woman has had her uterus removed.

PAGET'S DISEASE

Paget's disease is far less common than osteoporosis but is more likely to be noticed because it is easily recognizable on an X-ray and causes more obvious physical changes. Sometimes the first clue to its presence shows up in a blood test called *alkaline phosphatase*, which is one of the routine screening blood tests your doctor may order.

Unlike osteoporosis, where the bone is weaker but still normally formed, the construction of bone in Paget's disease proceeds in an erratic way. Normally, the inner mesh of bone is woven as symmetrically as a fine tapestry. In Paget's disease it is spun in total disarray, probably because it is spun too quickly. Even though the calcium cement is deposited normally, the bone loses its normal strength and resiliency because the underlying mesh is weak.

In Paget's disease, the bone may appear abnormal on X-ray but it rarely causes symptoms. As we have said, the condition is more than likely to be discovered by accident or while you are being tested for some other problem.

Where symptoms are present, they can vary from vague aches to marked deformity of bone. Softer bones may buckle under the weight of the body or even from the constant pull of muscles. For example, the shinbones may bend forward or the thighbones arch sideways. One of the more striking changes occurs in the skull bones. In most cases all the person will notice is a gradual increase in his hat size. More unusually, the changes may become apparent to others as the upper skull and forehead enlarge, as though the dome of the head were rising like dough. In extreme cases, the expanding bone, like the leading edge of an advancing glacier, may begin to slowly press against certain nerves in the skull. The nerves for hearing lie directly in the path of this growing bone and are usually the first to be affected, resulting in some hearing loss. Other nerves may ultimately become entrapped, but this is distinctly rare.

Just about any bone in the body can be affected by Paget's disease. It is often first noticed in the pelvic bone on X-ray but is unlikely to cause any symptoms there. Like osteoporosis, Paget's disease can weaken the building blocks of the spine, the vertebrae, and cause their collapse, resulting in back pains.

TREATMENT OF PAGET'S DISEASE

Few people ever develop serious problems from Paget's disease. The worst that they experience is minor pains, especially in the back and legs. Aspirin will usually suffice for these. Only rarely will something stronger be necessary. Still, if you know you have this condition, you must be cautious and avoid those obvious occasions that invite accidents. We have outlined some of these above in discussing osteoporosis.

Active investigation into the cause and treatment of Paget's disease has been continuing for a number of years. Several newer approaches to the treatment of this condition have grown out of this work. A few of these are now used for more severe cases.

One treatment that appears to be safe and easy to use is diphosphonate. Pain is often much relieved after several weeks' use. It is convenient to use since it can be taken by mouth.

Another effective medication is calcitonin. This is a hormone, derived from the thyroid gland, and must be given by injection. Not only will it result in significant relief of pain but it may actually halt the manufacture of abnormal bone. Unfortunately, not everyone responds equally well to this drug. Moreover, it is still not clear how long treatment remains effective.

The most potent form of therapy is a drug called mithramycin. Since this is a powerful drug with many side effects, it is reserved for people with the worst forms of Paget's disease. Few cases will call for the use of this drug.

THE SPINE

At one point in evolution, one of our adventurous ancestors decided to walk upright, thus freeing his arms for other uses. No doubt one of his first primitive words were the Neanderthal equivalent of "Oh, my aching back." For, with the upright posture, the weight of the body that previously had been equally distributed on four limbs now had to be supported by the lower back. Though the language may have changed down through time, the complaints remain the same.

The spinal column is a marvel of refined simplicity, perfectly engineered for the complicated role it must perform. It is composed of a series of bony blocks, called vertebrae, stacked upon one another and linked by outstretched bony arms. Snugly wedged between each vertebra is a tough flexible cushion, called the *disc* (fig. 28), which acts as a shock absorber. The entire chain of vertebrae and discs are firmly fastened together by taut bindings called *ligaments* and buttressed on either side by powerful muscles. These muscles enable us to perform demanding feats of strength while keeping the spine firmly moored in place. All the weight the spine bears pivots on a narrow area at the end of the spine like a flagpole on its base. This area is called the *sacrum* (fig. 27), and it is located in the small of the back. If this weren't enough, the constant buffeting from the lower part of our body is also aimed directly on this area, because the sacrum also joins with the pelvic bone. This junction is referred to as the *sacroiliac* area. Distress here is so common that just about everyone knows that sacroiliac pain means back pain. If you think about it, it is remarkable how little difficulty our spine gives us. Certainly, supporting our body seems simple enough. After all, a solitary tree trunk withstands the weight of many swaying branches. But we are

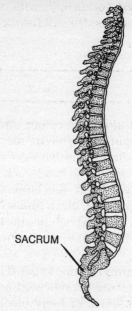

SACRUM

Fig. 27   Spinal column.

not planted in one spot. We walk, bend, turn, and lift. The greenest sapling would snap at the arch turned by the gymnast's back. Sturdy supports would buckle under the heavy load the stevedore must bear. Even though most of us don't put our backs to such extreme tests, our everyday activities make extraordinary demands on the spine.

CAUSE OF BACK PAIN

No one has to be told how painful a backache can be. The problem is that most backaches feel alike whether due to a serious problem or a minor sprain. Back pain can be misleading if the cause has nothing to do with the spine. For example, back pain can be prominent in problems related to the kidneys, pancreas, prostate, female reproductive organs, or even an enlarging blood vessel in the abdomen (aortic aneurysm). For this reason any new back pain that persists should be checked out with your doctor.

In the overwhelming majority of cases, however, the source of the trouble will be the spinal column or its supporting structures. In fact, the common backache we all experience most often arises in the ligaments and muscles that keep the spine firmly braced. In older people, the cushioning discs begin to shrink and muscles lose some of their strength and firm elasticity, and are more easily overtaxed. When they are injured by overstretching, the condition is called a *sprain*. Overexertion or inflammation can cause spasm of the muscles of the spine, another common cause of severe backache.

Often there is an obvious explanation for the back pain: too much lifting or strenuous activity. On the other hand, back pain can be a recurrent, nagging complaint, appearing intermittently over the years. This can be frustrating, leading to fruitless visits to the doctor and an endless battery of X-ray examinations. The problem is that while X-rays and their newer computerized versions (CAT scan) can tell us a great deal about the bony spine, they cannot examine the ligaments or muscles of our spine. These remain hidden from the most sophisticated diagnostic tests, but not from the sufferer. If your doctor seems to be ordering too many tests that have nothing to do with the spine, he's only being thorough. Keep in mind that many conditions outside of the spine can resemble back pain.

Don't be surprised or upset if, in the end, your doctor can't find anything definite to account for your distress. This happens quite often. It doesn't mean that your pain is not real. We just don't have the means available yet to diagnose every cause of back pain. Nevertheless, effective measures are available to handle this common problem.

WHAT TO DO ABOUT BACK PAIN

Never ignore a back pain that persists for several weeks. Find out what the problem is. If your doctor assures you that nothing is seriously wrong, here are a few things that may be useful to keep in mind.

  1. Avoid strain on your back. This means no lifting and frequent rest. Move cautiously so you won't find yourself

making a sudden back-wrenching bend or inadvertent backward turn.

2. Ask your doctor about some of the simple exercises to strengthen the support structures of your spine.

3. A heating pad or hot water bottle can go a long way in soothing the spasm of tense muscles when the pain is very severe.

4. Keep your weight under control. Remember, every pound you gain is an additional burden on your back.

5. Try a hard mattress or bed board on your bed. This helps keep the spine straight and reduces undue strain on the ligaments.

6. Find out whether a back brace or girdle would be of value to you. Your doctor should be able to let you know whether there are any disadvantages in your case.

7. Sometimes an electrostimulator provides surprising relief, although we do not know exactly how it does this. Again, your doctor is the best person to decide whether you might benefit from this kind of treatment.

8. Stick to the mildest type of pain reliever. Your back may give you trouble intermittently, and you don't want to become accustomed to strong medication.

ARTHRITIS OF SPINE

The common effects of the ordinary wear and tear of living are nowhere more apparent than in the spine. The same condition, osteoarthritis (see page 212), that bruises our joints is even more likely to affect our spines where the effects of time and wear are concentrated and magnified. All of us will eventually show some traces of osteoarthritis but few of us will ever be aware of it. In some cases, the bones become frosted with new bony growths, called *osteophytes*. Because the spinal cord, nerves, and vertebrae are so close to one another, these iciclelike projections from the vertebrae can occasionally nudge too close to a nerve from the spine. This can lead to back pain and even shooting pains remote from the spine, as down the arms, neck, or back of the leg. Usually proper rest, heat, and a properly fitting corset or neck brace will relieve the symptoms. Caution: Don't treat

yourself or act upon the advice of friends. Let your doctor
decide what treatment best suits your problem.

The other bone conditions that we have previously discussed (osteoporosis and Paget's disease, see pages 228, 232)
frequently affect the spine. Since osteoporosis is a normal
part of growing old, we come to expect a minor degree in the
spine also. In most cases this does not lead to any problem

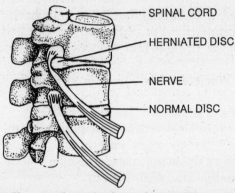

Fig. 28   Close-up of spinal column showing herniated disc pinching nerve.

and should be no cause for concern in most people, but occasionally can cause severe pain. For the most part, the measures outlined earlier apply to this condition as well. The
same holds true for Paget's disease.

SLIPPED DISC

The tough flexible cushion nestled between each of the vertebrae is called the *intervertebral disc* or *disc* for short. It
has a hard outer layer and a softer core. This inner core is
well encased and adds a certain degree of resiliency and
bounce to the disc, just as springs do to a car. This gummy
core may be squeezed out if a tear occurs in the outer covering of the disc. It is this escaped core that is referred to as
the *slipped disc*, presumably meaning that it has "slipped
out." Another word meaning exactly the same is *herniated
disc*. The spinal column, the spinal cord, and its nerves share

a very limited space and lie very close to one another. As the firm center of the disc is squeezed out, it is likely to encounter one of the nerves of the spinal cord (see Fig. 28). Symptoms from pressure on this nerve will vary depending on the level of the spine where the slipped disc occurs. Most slipped discs are found in the lower back. Pressure on nerves in this region may lead to low back pain as well as shooting pains or numbness down the back or side of the leg. On occasion, the pain can be quite deceptively limited to a small area, as for example around the knee joint or hip, simulating arthritis. Even weakness of a leg can develop. If the region of the spine involved by a disc is located in the neck, pain may shoot to the shoulder or down the arm or hand. In any event, symptoms can be quite subtle, ranging from "pins and needles" sensations to gripping, electric shocklike pain.

Your doctor may often suspect the condition simply by your description of the pain, or your recalling a specific event that was tied in with the onset of the pain, such as heavy lifting. After careful examination, he may decide to treat you with simple measures or seek to clarify the situation with more complicated tests. One of the simpler tests called an *electromyogram* (or EMG) measures the electrical conduction of nerves and muscle. To localize the site of the disc precisely, it may be necessary to perform a special X-ray called a *myelogram*. After injection of a small amount of dye into the spinal canal, it is possible for an X-ray to detect any pressure or blockage on the spinal cord. With the help of these and other techniques, such as the CAT Scan, it is possible to accurately diagnose and localize the source of the problem.

Treatment of Slipped Disc

The object of treatment is to reduce the inflammation caused by irritation from pressure on the nerve root by the fleshy slipped disc. To achieve this, the individual must eliminate all weight bearing on the spine by strict bed rest for a few days to a few weeks. During this time, application of local heat to relieve muscle spasm as well as use of pain relievers may be necessary. In special cases, it may be necessary to keep the spine perfectly aligned and immobile by traction. But usually bed rest will be enough to relieve the pain and pressure on the nerves.

If simple measures fail or if serious nerve injury develops, the most satisfactory approach is to remove by surgery the crabmeat-like disc causing nerve compression. The operation is usually quite successful.

A method of treatment that has not gained wide acceptance in this country but that still has enthusiastic support here and particularly in some other countries involves injecting certain enzymes (chymopapain) into the herniated disc in an effort to dissolve it. An extensive study in this country has shown that the method is no more effective than injecting simple pain relievers into the area. Nevertheless, some people are so fearful of surgery, no matter how safe, that they are willing to try any other method. This technique is inadvisable because of its many potentially severe side effects. There is no single best method of treatment for disc disease. Conservative treatment or surgery has been proven to be equally effective methods of treatment, depending on the situation that will be judged on an individual basis by your doctor.

SUMMARY

1. Our bones, like the rest of us, inevitably feel the wear and tear of time. Most of us, however, have nothing more than minor aches or pains.

2. Back pain is the price we pay for being able to walk upright. Most back pain is due to tension on muscles and ligaments but on occasion, the bony blocks or the spinal disc may be the source.

3. Never ignore any back pain that is persistent.

4. Not all back pain comes from the spine. Other conditions may reveal themselves as back pain.

5. There is no single best treatment for the problem of back pain regardless of its cause. Conservative therapy remains the best method of treatment unless serious nerve injury requires further action.

16

SEX—
GOOD AT ANY AGE

For the past twenty years, America has been through a sexual revolution. And, from all present signs, it isn't over yet. For most of our people, the revolution has helped to open up bedroom secrets to scientific observation and inquiry. But the taboo against sexual interest and activity in the elderly is still quite strong. And the stereotypes of the "dirty old man" and "has-been past her prime" are still with us. Sexual interest in the elderly is still the target of censure and ridicule by children, grandchildren, and others who typically disapprove with the old familiar refrain: "You're too old for that sort of thing." Why the taboo? Why the ridicule?

EXPOSING SOME MYTHS

American culture of the 1970s was dominated by a celebration of youth. Ours is the "Pepsi generation" where camaraderie, happiness, and, yes, even sex seem to belong exclusively to the young and the beautiful. Our young people and, indeed, our society as a whole have fostered the myth that sex is only for the young and that for those past sixty-five, sex is unbecoming, if not downright obscene and ridiculous.

Another factor that has contributed to the taboo against sex in the elderly is the nature of the "hang-ups" of professionals who serve and care for our older citizens. These young professionals—doctors, psychologists, social workers, and nurses—still harbor Victorian attitudes about the experiences of sex for those of their parents' generation. Their older clients tend to remind them of their own elderly parents. Having somewhat difficult problems contemplating their parents engaged in sexual activity, they experience similar problems accepting and dealing with the sexual activity of their older patients and even greater problems discussing them frankly and openly. Thus, until recently, the whole area of sexual function and behavior in the aging has remained shrouded in myth and ignorance.

Thanks to the early work of Kinsey and the more recent work of Masters and Johnson and other researchers, we have learned that sexual capacity is with us until very late in life. Sexual activity may change as we grow older but it certainly does not end.

Older women past menopause lose little of their sexual function. The aging woman's capacity to engage in sexual intercourse and to reach orgasm lasts as long as life itself. Though the vaginal area may be less lubricated because of a diminished output of estrogen, an application of a jelly or estrogen cream or other lubricant promotes intercourse without discomfort. Orgasm may take longer to achieve and may become shorter in duration and intensity. The important point is that for most women it can be achieved.

This continued sexual vitality is especially likely to continue in postmenopausal women who were sexually active in their younger and middle years. There is absolutely no basis for the old wives' tale that you can "wear it out" by overuse.

The sexual life of men is complicated by significant physiological changes that accompany aging. Achieving an erection takes longer, perhaps five to ten minutes, with tactile stimulation. Since there is a reduction in the volume of seminal fluid, the need to ejaculate decreases and may occur only once in two or three sessions of lovemaking. In addition, the refractory period, that is the time it takes after ejaculation for a man to have another erection and climax, increases, usually to more than twenty-four hours. These physiological changes, as upsetting as they may seem to an aging male, do not in any sense signify an end to sexual activity and satisfaction. Just as with women, the more sexually active a man has been through his early and middle years, the more sexually vital he will be as he grows older.

A recent study by the Duke University Center for the Study of Aging and Human Development has given us astounding statistics about sexual function in older men—despite their physiological changes. Out of over one hundred subjects with an average age of sixty-eight, 70 percent were still sexually active. After ten years, with average age of seventy-eight, the proportion had dropped to 25 percent. Though the decline in proportion was great, still, at age seventy-eight, one in four men were still sexually vital, a greater proportion than most people had believed. And for a small but significant proportion of the original sample, sexual expression actually increased over a ten-year period.

Nature works in strange and sometimes wondrous ways. The physiological changes that occur in men and women appear to help rather than hinder the sexual compatibility of aging couples. Though the man needs even more time to become aroused and ejaculate, the woman needs more time to become lubricated, attain clitoral stimulation, and reach orgasm. In fact, some women past fifty have reported a greater likelihood of reaching orgasm during intercourse as their mates require more time for arousal and climax. The more sexual interest and pleasure they share during the early and middle years, the more they will have in their later years.

IMPOTENCE

Every doctor is familiar with the man who comes to him complaining that it takes him longer to get an erection than

it used to. Sometimes he cannot get an erection at all, he
cannot achieve satisfactory orgasm, he cannot have intercourse as frequently as he used to. "What is happening to
me, Doc?" he asks. "Can I do anything about it? Am I becoming impotent?"

The simple, inescapable fact is that something indeed is
happening to him. He is just getting older and certain
changes are taking place in him. He can't do all the things he
used to do, not as frequently, and not as zestfully. But
chances are he is not impotent. His sexual life is not finished.
It is just changing with the oncoming years.

PSYCHOLOGICAL FACTORS

Contrary to popular belief, the cause of sexual impotence in
males is psychological in ninety out of one hundred cases.
Though physiological changes are taking place and will continue to take place, these changes do not mean that the older
man must close the curtain on sexual fulfillment. What happens is that by watching and worrying about the gradual
slowing up of his sexual functioning, he becomes alarmed
as he imagines he is losing all of his former "male powers."
With alarm comes anxiety and tension, even depression. As
he fails at his next attempt at intercourse, his fears and depression deepen. What he had most feared has happened.
He has become temporarily impotent for reasons that are
both physical and psychological. Ironically, the impotence
he had feared has been brought on by deepening fear itself.
While the physiological changes he has noticed in his sexual
functioning may have triggered the fear, they did not produce impotence.

SUCCESS OF COUNSELING

What can be done for the temporarily impotent male?
Counseling by a urologist has proven extremely effective in
bolstering a man's view of himself. The urologist can, in
most instances, assure him that he is not "over the hill." The
attention and the emotional support of the urologist quiets
the man's many fears in as few as three or four office visits. If

the man has a willing and understanding partner, such uro-
logic counseling proves successful about 60 percent of the
time.

Needless to say, not all urologists are capable of providing the kind of sympathy and support needed for successful
counseling. Some are unsure about their own sexuality or too
inhibited to discuss the matter openly. So the individual
should not always assume that lack of communication is *his*
fault. He should ask to be referred to another urologist. The
doctor should grant this request without hesitation.

Other kinds of therapy for impotence have also proved
effective. Masters and Johnson's intensive retraining therapy
and Helen Kaplan's "new sex therapy" have high success
rates for patients who have not gotten anywhere by talking
to their doctors. Many other forms of successful therapy are
available. Some therapists use hypnosis; others use small
doses of barbiturates to relax their patients. All these treatments are beneficial provided that the man experiences a
reasonably rapid return of his sexual interest and fulfillment.

The treatment of impotence through the taking of male
hormones is not considered desirable. First, there is no scientific evidence that it really works. Second, there is some
evidence that such hormone therapy may increase your
chances of developing cancer of the prostate and having
problems with your heart.

PHYSICAL CAUSES OF IMPOTENCE

Though the vast majority of impotent males become so because of fear and depression, approximately 10 percent of
impotence is due to physical problems. Before discussing
these physical disorders, we must understand how an erection normally occurs. The penis is made up of large blood
vessels that can hold a great deal of blood. It is the blood
filling these vessels that hardens the penis during erection.
The stimulation of certain nerves coming from the lower
spine (sacral plexus) is required to open these blood vessels
so that the blood can enter.

All the physical causes of impotence affect either these

nerves or blood vessels: (1) Hardening of the arteries prevents sufficient blood from reaching the penis. (2) Surgery in the pelvic or rectal area destroys the key nerves. (3) Certain medications, especially those given for hypertension, sometimes paralyze these nerves. (4) Diabetes mellitus damages the nerves and causes hardening of the arteries. Since diabetes and hypertension are so common, it is fair to assume that the majority of physically impotent men are either diabetic or being treated for hypertension.

If impotence is caused by drugs, it is easily correctible. Tell your doctor and he may change your present medication to one without this undesirable side effect.

Unfortunately, other causes of impotence are not so easily eliminated. Occasionally, surgery to bypass a blockage in an artery (hypogastric artery) in the lower abdomen can alleviate impotence caused by hardening of the arteries. The results of this operation, however, have only been fair. An arteriogram (see page 11) is necessary to demonstrate the block if surgery is contemplated.

Although most physically caused impotence cannot be reversed, partial sexual satisfaction for both the impotent man and his partner may be possible with the use of various artificial devices that can be attached to the penis. Your physician can refer you to a urologist who can fit you for such a device.

IS SEX A PHYSICAL STRAIN?

It is well known that pulse rate, blood pressure, and rate of breathing increase with sexual excitement. These physiological changes are linked to emotional excitement during the sex act, not to the sexual function itself. The actual sexual activity requires no more energy than does a brisk walk at a rate of two to two and one-half miles per hour or perhaps a climb up one flight of steps.

Regular intercourse with a familiar partner of many years does not lead to undue emotional excitement and is not likely to be threatening to the health of either partner. On the other hand, cardiac insufficiency and, occasionally, sudden death may occur in older men who engage in illicit lovemaking where the emotional climate is usually quite intense.

SEX AFTER A HEART ATTACK?

Many men are afraid of having sex after a heart attack. If you have recovered sufficiently to take a brisk walk or climb a flight of steps, you are probably ready for sex. Check with your doctor. Chances are that eight to fourteen weeks after your attack he will let you gradually resume sexual activity, provided you have made an uncomplicated recovery.

One recommendation for sexual activity in cardiac patients is a change in the male's position during the sex act. If the male is in the traditional position above the woman, intercourse will require use of arm and chest muscles that are not necessary to the sex act itself. If he changes to a position beneath his partner, he does not need to use those muscles and hence requires less energy during the sex act. Of course, this kind of change in lifelong habits is not easy. But it can be achieved if both partners are sensitive and understanding.

THE PROBLEMS OF WOMEN

Unlike men, limitations of sexual activity in women are rarely physical. Although older woman may develop some vaginal atrophy (thinning of the membrane of the vagina), application of a jelly or estrogen cream usually corrects the condition.

While the physical problems of female sexual dysfunction can be easily overcome, the majority of older women still do not fulfill their potential for sexual enjoyment. There are complex social and psychological reasons for this.

First, the sexual needs of women of all ages have long

been misunderstood. A woman's sexual response, or lack thereof, can easily be hidden from her partner. Traditionally, a woman came to bed to conceive and bear children and to fulfill her partner's needs. Her own needs were of secondary or no importance.

Happily, the special sexual needs of women are now better understood. We know now that most women are unable to reach orgasm without tactile stimulation of the clitoral region. It is stimulation of the clitoris, not the vagina, to which women respond during foreplay and intercourse. If a male partner does not know this, or if a woman is too inhibited to tell him, the woman will remain unfulfilled and unsatisfied during and after intercourse.

If older women are to fulfill their potential for sexual enjoyment, they must better understand the needs of their own bodies and then communicate those needs to their partners.

The social and cultural pressures that inhibit sexual fulfillment are formidable, indeed. At age sixty-five, the ratio of men to women is 129 women for every 100 men. By age seventy-five, the ratio is 156 women for every 100 men. More significant even than this ratio is the fact that most men of sixty-five or older are married while more than half the women in the same age range are unmarried. It is not unusual to find, in a housing project for the elderly, as few as two available men for as many as two hundred women. The lack of a socially acceptable sexual partner unfortunately puts an end to sexual activity in women who still remain sexually vital, physically and emotionally.

Unhappily, the double standard still exists. For elderly men, being married or unmarried does not affect their sexual interest and activity. For elderly women, however, marriage is everything, for it is rare for a woman born before 1920 to engage in sexual activity with a partner to whom she is not married. There are some strong signs, however, that the coming generations of liberated women will put an end to the double standard.

SEX AND THE ELDERLY: SOME FINAL WORDS

What about the social pressures on couples? Many elderly people have no choice but to live with their middle-aged children who often feel that their parents are too old for "that sort of thing." Lack of privacy and a fear of seeming ridiculous in the eyes of insensitive children and grandchildren frequently causes estrangement and the end of sexual intimacy. So, older couples must retain their independence and live in their own homes as long as possible.

For the single elderly person, the problem is even greater. Social service centers provide adequate recreation for daytime hours. But the long evenings bring only loneliness. Remarriage can be emotionally and socially satisfying and should be encouraged if the couple share common interests and values. There is some evidence that remarriage extends the likelihood of longer life for both partners. And contrary to common belief, second marriages are most successful among those who have had healthy, sexually satisfying first marriages.

Many of our elderly cannot live with their children, cannot remarry, and fail to "make it" on their own. For these, approximately 5 percent, there exists the vast proliferation of nursing homes or adult homes. As with all long-term care facilities, the environment becomes easily dehumanized and, of course, desexualized. Wards are traditionally segregated and the bed check every two hours hardly encourages meaningful, fulfilling sexual activity.

Certainly, most of the elderly living in nursing homes are no longer sexually interested or active. But for those who are, there is a basic denial of their rights as human beings.

Our American way of aging—living with son or daughter or in an adult home—stands in sharp contrast to the way other nations have handled the same problem. In England and the Scandinavian countries, subsidized housing is available to the elderly in planned villages. Here the privacy of independent apartment dwelling is encouraged. The apartments are architecturally designed to enable people, even those with physical infirmities, to stay in their own homes as long as possible. At the same time the needs of the lonely and infirm are met through communal dining and recreational facilities. Doctors, nurses, and therapists are readily available when needed. Here the freedom to realize one's sexual potential is preserved while other needs, both social and medical, are cared for. We have much to learn from the English and Scandinavians.

SUMMARY

Age is no barrier to the enjoyment of sex:

1. Women are capable of fully enjoying sex long after their menopause. In fact, older women often experience more complete orgasm than they did when they were younger.

2. Sometimes, vaginal glands may dry up in older women, but this can be corrected with jellies or estrogen creams.

3. Very few men become impotent for physical reasons as they grow older. Impotence is more often caused by fear or depression. After a good examination to rule out physical causes of impotence, psychological support may be helpful.

4. Male hormone injections do not relieve impotence and are dangerous.

5. Older couples are entitled to the same privacy as younger people. It is lack of privacy or a suitable mate that often leads to the end of an older person's sexuality. Given the appropriate partner, sexuality can last as long as life itself.

17

CHANGES
IN PERSONALITY

Many people assume that older people cannot think clearly simply because they are older. This point of view is unfortunately not confined to laymen. It is quite prevalent among people in the medical field. In fact, we sometimes feel that acquaintances, relatives, and friends often treat elderly people with more respect than many social workers, doctors, and nurses do. These professionals who should know better, attribute the older person's apparent slowness of movement and response to declining intellect. They couldn't be more wrong.

It is true that the brain, like all other organs of the body, is affected by the aging process and gradually loses some of its sharpness. Beyond the age of forty, there is gradual loss of the nerve cells (neurons) involved in thinking and memory. The very brightest of us become less creative and less able to think on the very highest levels. Theoretical physicists often complete their most creative work by the age of forty. A review of the achievements of Nobel laureates in chemistry and physics demonstrates this trend, too. However, for most of us who have never functioned on this lofty plane, changes in our intellectual capacity are usually not apparent to us or to others. It has been estimated that we use only a very small percentage of our nerve cells in our lifetime, and so our reserve supply is enormous.

CHANGES WITH AGE

In many cases, it is difficult to determine why aging brings
with it certain changes. But we feel pretty sure that psychological and personality factors play a major role. Not all
elderly people develop these changes. Many retain not only
a great deal of their youthful vigor but they also radiate a
zest for life and a boldness of spirit. People with a positive,
outgoing, optimistic attitude in their early years are more
likely to be relaxed, flexible, and confident in their later
years. Unfortunately, however, many more people tend to
move in other, less positive directions. Getting older inevitably changes our personalities, our ways of thinking and be-
having, sometimes noticed only by our children and spouses.
What are these changes? How can we recognize them and
what can we do to help older people? What can they do to
help themselves?

SLOWER RESPONSE

In the course of conversation, older people often respond
more slowly to questions and remarks. Sometimes this apparently slower response is simply the result of the deeper
reflection, greater maturity, and richer experiences that the
older person brings to bear on a subject. He may see fewer
absolutes and more shades of right and wrong than his
younger counterpart who responds more quickly. In some
instances, however, the older person cannot think as quickly
as he used to because his reflexes are slowing up. In part,
this is due to the fact that older nerves cannot carry messages to the brain as quickly as younger ones.

RIGIDITY

Older people naturally find it difficult to change their personal habits, attitudes, and behavior. They find quick
changes of plans and new ways of doing things bothersome
and somewhat frightening. This inability or unwillingness to
change probably reflects a loss of confidence in one's ability

to handle oneself, to think quickly, and to protect oneself. Older people often insist on leading a controlled life, planning each activity well in advance, and thus avoiding tension and anxiety.

Strong characteristics of an individual's personality when he was younger tend to become exaggerated and stand out prominently as he grows older. For example, a frugal person may become stingy; a hypochondriac may be virtually paralyzed by fear of poor health; an introverted person may become almost a hermit. In some instances, it is as though the whole personality were frozen into a block of ice unable to bend or sway with everyday experiences.

MEMORY

With most people, one function of the mind tends to weaken with advanced age: memory. Curiously, the older person often has no difficulty remembering things long past. He can tell you in great detail about scenes from his childhood and even events that happened a few years ago. His difficulty is usually with recent memory, particularly of events that happened within the last few days or weeks. The reason for this difference is to be found in the way the brain works. Old memory areas, once established, hold up quite well unless destroyed by a disease process. On the other hand, recent memory is rather loosely held in the brain. If it is not processed into the old memory areas, it will be lost. This ability of the brain to transfer newly remembered events into the old memory areas is gradually impaired with age.

SEVERE CHANGES

The personality changes that we have described as a normal part of aging develop very gradually. On the other hand, if you notice marked changes in behavior, personality, or intellectual capacity over a short period in a friend or relative, what should you do? First, determine whether his unusual behavior can be a result of stresses, tensions, or family problems. It may be appropriate for someone to show frustration and anger about unpleasant circumstances in his life. The solution is probably not medical. Solving his problem may require social workers, family counselors, or financial experts. If there is no obvious reason for the change in his behavior, mood, or thinking, see a doctor.

The doctor's first job is to determine whether these changes are organic or functional. By this we mean: Are they caused by some specific disease (organic) in the brain or are they purely psychological (functional) in nature? The doctor must try to obtain as complete a history as possible of the events leading up to the present symptoms. If the patient cannot supply this information, the doctor must speak to a close friend or relative. The doctor must also perform a complete neurological examination, looking especially for any so-called focal signs such as weakness in an arm or leg, facial sag, garbled speech, visual problems, or loss of sensation. These signs usually point to some physical cause of the abnormal behavior.

The most important part of the doctor's examination is evaluation of the patient's mental status. Basically, he checks four mental functions: orientation, memory, general knowledge, and intellectual capacity. By orientation, we mean knowing who you are, where you are, and what month and year you are in. If a person cannot answer these questions accurately, he is disoriented, a sign that his brain is not working well.

MEMORY TESTING

The examination of memory requires a check on both recent and past events. As we have pointed out, it is normal for older people to have some difficulty in remembering recent events. An older person should be able to remember the broad outlines of his past (even his childhood), his social relationships, and his recent daily activities. For example, we should be concerned if he can't remember his address, names of children, or major daily activities.

On the other hand, it is not unusual for older people to be unable to remember the details of a conversation they had a few days ago. They may tell the same anecdotes and jokes every few weeks to the same people. They may also find it more difficult to remember the names of new acquaintances or travel directions. None of these lapses should be any cause for alarm.

TESTING GENERAL KNOWLEDGE

The testing of general knowledge is really an examination of both memory and concentration. For example, the doctor may ask the individual to identify the president of the United States, vice-president, governor, mayor, and other elected officials, and to discuss current events in general. Or he may ask about his hobbies and cultural interests. Here it is very important for the doctor to know something about his patient's past interests, generally inquiring in some depth and detail about subjects especially interesting to him. For example, the doctor would question an avid baseball fan about teams, players, and rules of the game. He would expect a gardener to speak clearly about flowers but would not be surprised if he showed no interest in baseball. Questions like these and the answers they evoke may give the doctor some idea as to whether an individual is losing his memory and ability to put his thoughts together, or is just becoming uninterested in his surroundings. The doctor here is trying to distinguish between an organic brain problem and a psychological depression.

Finally, the doctor will want to check the individual's intellectual capacity. Can he interpret proverbs? Can he answer commonsense questions? Can he perform simple arithmetical calculations? Can he repeat a series of numbers spoken to him? Can he repeat them in reversed order? All of these questions and many others can give the doctor some idea of intellectual capacity. But he must be very careful in drawing conclusions from these mental tests. It is impossible to know with certainty how much intellectual loss any individual has suffered without knowing a good deal about his previous abilities. In some instances, the loss is obvious. If the doctor knows that the patient was not mentally retarded as a child, he can assume that his failure to do very simple calculations or to recite three-digit numbers accurately points to a serious problem. However, an uneducated, simple person may never have been able to interpret proverbs or do fourth-grade arithmetical problems.

In some individuals, the degree of loss may be underestimated. Someone unusually gifted with certain skills may still perform them acceptably when he is not able to do other things. For example, an accountant may perform arithmetical calculations correctly even though other tests would show wide gaps in his thinking ability. He will have to lose many nerve cells before he forgets how to do arithmetic because he started out on a very high level. For this reason, the doctor's questions must touch on many areas of ordinary daily life to get a rounded, composite picture of a person's abilities.

IS THE PROBLEM ORGANIC OR PSYCHOLOGICAL?

In most cases, the detailed neurological and mental testing will enable the doctor to decide whether his patient has some sort of brain disease or is suffering from psychological problems. But even after thorough testing and evaluation, he cannot always be sure he has made the right diagnosis. Psychological depression, for example, can make a person seem mentally dull. The depressed person may not respond well to questions because he cannot focus his attention on his environment. Labeling such a depressed person as senile would be a great mistake, one that unfortunately doctors sometimes make, no matter how careful they are. A clue to depression may be the changing nature of his responses. At times, he may converse appropriately and, at other times, he may not answer any questions at all. Here, the history of his behavior obtained from a close friend or relative may be critically important. For a fuller discussion of symptoms of depression, see page 260.

Following intensive interviewing, the doctor may obtain a brain wave test (*electroencephalogram* or EEG) if he still is unsure whether the problem is organic or psychological. In this simple test, the electrical waves transmitted from the brain are recorded. In the overwhelming majority of cases, the brain wave test will show clear-cut abnormalities if there is an organic brain problem. Therefore, a normal EEG suggests a psychological explanation for changes in behavior.

CAUSES OF BRAIN PROBLEMS

If the individual does have evidence of brain problems, his doctor must attempt to establish the cause. As we have pointed out in previous chapters, the brain depends on proper functioning of many other areas of the body to maintain its own health. It must receive oxygen and nutrition, and so there must be an adequate circulation and sufficient red blood cells to carry oxygen. The brain is also very sensitive to harmful substances. It is not surprising then that the loss of intellectual ability has many causes:

1. *Heart problems* (including heartbeat and rhythm)
2. *Circulation problems* (clogged arteries to the brain)
3. *Anemia* (too few red blood cells to carry oxygen)
4. *Hypoglycemia* (low blood-sugar level)
5. *Kidney problems* with accumulation of waste products
6. *Liver problems* with accumulation of ammonia and other poisons
7. *Lung problems* with lack of oxygen and accumulation of carbon dioxide in the blood
8. *Hypothyroidism*
9. *Overusage* of tranquilizer and sleeping medications
10. *Poor hearing and poor vision*, leading to sensory deprivation
11. *Problems in the brain itself.*

A doctor faced with a person suffering from mental changes must consider all these categories and conduct a thorough search for the cause. His goal is to find as many reversible factors as possible so that he can help his patient. If this search does not reveal any factors outside the brain, he must turn his attention to the brain itself.

A new technique called *computerized axial tomography* (CAT scan) has revolutionized the way we diagnose brain problems. In this test, a whole series of X-rays of different strengths are taken simultaneously from many different angles so that we actually get a picture of the entire brain. With this test, doctors can usually determine, for example, whether or not a brain tumor is present. Although brain tumors are relatively rare, they must be looked for because they are often curable by surgery in the early stages. A small tumor in the front of the brain may account for mental changes in behavior or thinking.

An even more important reason for doing a CAT scan is to make sure that we do not miss a condition called *normal pressure hydrocephalus* (water on the brain). There are a series of connecting cavities inside the brain and a fluid flows through them. If one of these cavities becomes blocked, fluid builds up and exerts pressure on the brain. This pressure gradually damages and destroys nerve cells.

In the last ten years, neurologists have found that normal pressure hydrocephalus may occur for unknown reasons in middle-aged and older people and lead to subtle mental deterioration. Many people considered senile may be suffering from this condition. Most important, something can be done to overcome this problem through special neurosurgery. A neurosurgeon can correct the blockage by inserting a tube into the blocked cavity and hooking it up to a vein in the neck. The fluid can then flow out of the cavities of the brain, and mental loss will cease. If this hydrocephalus is treated in an early stage, mental functions may improve.

If all the laboratory tests are negative, the mental loss is unfortunately the result of one of two incurable conditions. Either the individual is having a progressive series of small strokes or brain cells are being lost for unknown reasons. The former condition is due to *arteriosclerosis* (see Chapter 1) and the latter condition is called *senile dementia*. Unfortunately, this kind of progressive brain damage cannot be halted.

TREATING SENILITY

What can we do for a person with senile dementia or arteriosclerosis? It is essential not to permit him to withdraw from or to lose contact with people and activities that are important in his life. This contact can be maintained in an orderly, nontaxing way so that he is not overwhelmed by a bewildering array of persons and tasks that are now beyond his capacity. Elderly people frequently stop traveling on their own and lose contact with important friends, relatives, and activities because of increasing confusion, insecurity, and poor health. They can be given assistance and encouragement in maintaining these essential contacts as long as possible. If necessary, they should be encouraged to join social or recreational programs for the elderly. These activities provide substitute relationships and involvement when there is a substantial loss of relationships through death, retirement, or moving away from peers.

It is also important to provide external clues and support in order to fill in memory gaps. In this way, the senile individual is not confronted with the extent of his confusion. For example, a night light in the bedroom helps to avoid the increased bewilderment that occurs when he gets up at night to go to the bathroom. A wall clock provides constant feedback as to time and helps provide structure to the thinking process. The senile person can be tactfully told whom he is seeing and what will happen when he meets an individual he should know but does not remember. For example, one might say, "Cousin Joan Smith has come to visit you and take you out for a drive."

In many cases, senility is aggravated by poor vision, and/or poor hearing. Without proper sensory input, the confused individual becomes more confused. The elderly should have their vision and hearing checked regularly. Eyeglasses or a hearing aid may sometimes make a big difference in their alertness.

Adequate dental care including false teeth help older persons continue their usual dietary habits. This is not only important in maintaining nutritional status but also provides social outlets for the individual. They can join the family at mealtime.

Many older people are walking precariously on a fine line between total alertness and disorientation. If their surroundings are changed for more than a few days, they may lose their sense of time and place, especially at night. It is not uncommon for these people to become confused in the hospital if they wake up in the middle of the night. When they go home, they become perfectly alert again. These same people may also become confused if they get even a minor infection or fever. So never judge an older person's mental capacity or emotional condition when he is under stress or ill.

DEPRESSION

Depression is the chief psychological problem afflicting older people. This should come as no surprise because a significant percentage of our entire population suffers from depression at one time or another.

"Depression" is used by the lay public much too loosely. People often say that they are depressed whenever anything upsets them or makes them temporarily unhappy. But, when we speak of true depression in a medical sense, we mean a prolonged period of unhappiness associated with loss of enthusiasm and inability to function as before. A depressed person has difficulty in carrying out his normal activities, finds it hard to concentrate on what he is doing, so much so that he may not even look at or listen to you when you speak to him. He tends to mope and be uncommunicative. Depression results in loss of energy of all kinds. The depressed individual may complain of tiredness, weakness, insomnia, and loss of sexual desire. In the more serious stages, a depressed person may be unable to perform such simple activities of daily living as dressing and bathing. He may stop eating and drinking, and sometimes even die of dehydration. Of course, not too many people develop such serious, life-threatening symptoms, but millions go through spells of minor to moderate depression that may not even be noticed by anyone except a close relative. Fortunately, most depression sufferers recover on their own, although they tend to have repeated episodes.

KINDS OF DEPRESSION

There are really two kinds of depression: exogenous and endogenous. Exogenous depression is caused by events out of the person's control. If he loses a spouse or has serious business reverses, for example, he may become understandably and appropriately depressed. Endogenous depression, on the other hand, stems from problems, fears, or feelings within the individual himself.

Elderly people often suffer from a combination of these. Psychiatrists refer to their problems as involutional depression. Major factors that may make them melancholy have to do with waning physical power, an increasing feeling that they are on the decline with nothing positive to look forward to, loneliness, and boredom. Certain milestones along the way accentuate these feelings. Retirement, for example, may leave someone without an important life role. This, of course, is more likely to happen if the individual has no interests or hobbies of his own.

Another significant event is the death of a spouse. Bereavement that occurs in response to such a loss is particularly difficult for the elderly. There is a significant increase in physical illnesses and death occurring in the first year of widowhood for the elderly compared to other people of the same age and background. A great deal of family and community support and understanding is essential during this particularly vulnerable time.

Very often, an elderly person becomes depressed by real medical problems. He may interpret every minor problem as the beginning of a general decline in vigor. Sometimes, depression complicates a process of true mental deterioration. Someone losing his memory and mental acuity may be aware of his loss and naturally become very melancholy. This may set in motion a vicious circle: The depression further decreases his ability to interact with people and this loss of stimulation results in further mental deterioration.

SUICIDE

The most dire consequence of depression is, of course, suicide. Unfortunately, it is very difficult to know when someone is likely to take his own life. Usually the individual shows some signs of depression first, but the depression does not have to be severe. In fact, suicide is less likely in the very severe stages of depression because the individual usually doesn't have enough emotional strength to plan or execute such an act. The most dangerous time is often when he is beginning to recover and has the strength to contemplate suicide.

Many people are aware that suicide is a leading cause of death among teen-agers and young adults, but relatively few realize that suicide takes a heavy toll of the elderly, too. Although suicide attempts are far more common during the younger and middle years, successful suicides are more common in the elderly. Psychiatrists regard a suicide attempt in an older person as a most serious occurrence that requires active treatment and concern for the safety of the individual. It is *not* true that people who talk about suicide never do anything. Most people who attempt or commit suicide usually signal their pain or concern or hopelessness to their family, friends, or doctor in advance. This should be taken as a "cry for help."

TREATMENT OF DEPRESSION

One we recognize a person suffering from depression, what should we do? There are no hard and fast rules about treatment, but here are a few guidelines:

1. First of all, you must make sure that the diagnosis is correct. If you have a relative or friend who is acting depressed or listless, take him to a competent doctor.

2. Secondly, make sure that the depressed individual won't take his life. This can be very difficult to determine. As

we pointed out earlier, it is often the moderately depressed rather than seriously depressed person who contemplates suicide. Your family doctor, after talking to the patient, may decide that urgent psychiatric consultation or hospitalization is necessary.

3. Next, some sort of psychological therapy must be instituted. The emphasis in an older depressed individual should be pragmatic, dealing with the specific symptoms and depressing factors in the patient's life. Prolonged psychoanalysis is generally not appropriate. Depending on the severity and nature of the problem, these therapy sessions may be conducted by a family doctor, a psychiatrist, psychologist, psychiatric nurse, social worker, or geriatric counselor. For most people, this treatment takes place outside of any institution. It is important to explore the individual's concerns and fears and help him to deal with them. Depression is often the reaction to some loss to the individual such as loss of self-esteem in the family and community, loss of important social and love relationships, or loss of outlets for social, intellectual, and recreational activities through physical and mental disabilities and dysfunction. In general, the therapist must identify the events and circumstances that contributed to these losses and help him to restore or replace them or to change his perception of these losses and to accept them.

4. The right amount of occupational therapy and socialization is important. Although the patient must accept his real loss of vigor, he should not limit his activities because of unjustified fears. It is important to get him involved with people in activities so that he can use his faculties effectively. There are many possibilities: volunteer work in the community, development of hobbies, educational activities, social programs in "Y's" and Golden Age clubs, and scores of others.

5. The therapist must decide what the patient is capable of doing. Pressing someone to do what he is not able to do leads to frustration and deeper depression. Do not push your depressed friend or relative too far without first discussing the problem with a professional.

6. Through this depressive crisis, it is very important

for the person to have access to a steady, understanding friend or relative. A family member or close friend is ideal, but very often a doctor or social worker may play this role. Part of successful therapy depends on the depressed person's desire to please this person by following advice. Little by little, he becomes involved in activities and comes out of his isolation.

Antidepressant Medications

In recent years, a host of effective antidepressant medications (tricyclic compounds) have become available. These powerful drugs are useful in the treatment of severe depression, although they are not likely to cure it by themselves. They can bring a very depressed person to the point where he can respond to counseling and emotional support. They are particularly effective in endogenous depression. The mood-elevating effects of these drugs are usually not fully apparent for three to four weeks. In the meantime, the individual must receive psychological support and protection.

Unfortunately, the tricyclic drugs may have very serious side effects and should never be used for mild symptoms before trying other approaches. They are often responsible for arrhythmias of the heart and are potentially fatal. Elderly people are more susceptible to heart complications than the young, especially if they have a history of heart trouble. Furthermore, a depressed person may intentionally or accidentally take an overdose of these pills. Many deaths have already been reported from antidepressant medication. The doctor must check the patient's heart status and obtain an electrocardiogram before prescribing these pills.

In high doses, antidepressant medications can lead to serious brain complications including hallucinations, convulsions, and coma. Less serious but annoying side effects include dry mouth and difficulty in urinating.

Shock Treatment

When someone is severely depressed and unable to respond to guidance and support, it may be necessary to resort to more drastic kinds of treatment. One such therapy is electro-shock treatment. Results are often excellent and quick. With a few such treatments, many very seriously depressed people snap out of their doldrums quickly. Obviously, we consider use of electroshock treatment only for extremely depressed people. Following this treatment, the patient may be a little confused for a few weeks, but he generally recovers. How-ever, there is always a small danger of permanent brain in-jury. So electroshock should be used only as a last resort.

ANXIETY

Anxiety can hit the elderly as hard as depression can. Aging often brings with it fear and insecurity. Many older people compensate for insecurity by planning their activities care-fully and keeping to a rigid schedule. But others are either not in a position to do this or lack the enormous amount of mental discipline that this scheduling requires. They may become so anxious and agitated that they cannot function. They may act very much like depressed people, displaying lethargy, lack of interest in their surroundings, and in-somnia. In fact, the two problems of anxiety and depression are definitely related. They are, in many ways, opposite sides of the same coin, both reactions to fears associated with aging.

In addition to counseling and support, people suffering from anxiety generally need medication. The major tranqui-lizer drugs such as Thorazine, Mellaril, and Haldol can be extremely helpful. They calm the mind without causing sleepiness. The doctor must start his patient with a small dose, gradually building it up until the symptoms are re-lieved. People who are both depressed and anxious may ob-tain relief of all their symptoms with these drugs. Since they are much safer than antidepressant pills, the latter should never be given to a person with symptoms of both anxiety and depression until the tranquilizers have been tried first.

The major side effect of tranquilizers is a stiffening of muscles, leading to difficulty in moving and sometimes painful muscle spasms. The jaw may become rigid, making eating and speaking difficult. The individual may also develop tremors of his hands and feet. Fortunately, no permanent damage occurs since the rigidity and tremors fade quickly when the drug is stopped. The doctor can often prevent this side effect by being prudent in the doses he prescribes and including another kind of pill to prevent muscle rigidity.

High doses of tranquilizers may interfere with proper functioning of the brain. People receiving large amounts of these drugs may be confused and lethargic and have a dull, dazed appearance. They may become very depressed and practically immobile. The doctor must be very careful, in using these tranquilizers, to increase the dose slowly until his patient is reasonably calm. He must try to find a happy medium between relief of anxiety and onset of sedation.

Some people will develop annoying dryness of the mouth and men with large prostates may have difficulty in urinating while taking tranquilizers. Lowering of the dose may be necessary if these symptoms occur.

PARKINSON'S DISEASE

One area of the brain, called the *basal ganglia*, is particularly subject to a gradual wearing-out process as we age. The resulting disorder, Parkinson's disease, causes movement problems but rarely impairs thinking ability. The incidence of this disorder rises over the age of sixty.

If you develop Parkinson's disease, you may notice that your hands shake slightly when you are not moving them voluntarily. This is called a *tremor*. You may also find that you cannot move as smoothly as you once did. Your muscles may be a little rigid, causing you to change position slowly. You may have to begin walking gradually, and your pace may be slower. In severe Parkinson's disease, the tremor may be enough to interfere with fine motor activities, such as writing, and rigidity may seriously hamper walking and rising. People with severe Parkinson's disease are said to have "masklike faces" because the rigidity of the facial muscles prevents normal changes in facial expression. Fortunately, most people with Parkinson's disease do not have a serious problem. They may have a little tremor and notice some mild stiffness that does not interfere with their normal activities.

For those who do have severe Parkinson's disease, there is now very effective medicine that can alleviate much of the problem. Researchers have found that Parkinson's disease occurs because of a deficiency of a chemical that transmits messages between nerve cells in the basal ganglia. The cells that normally make this chemical (dopamine) have worn out. A medication called L-Dopa can be taken by mouth, and the brain converts it to dopamine. Many previously immobilized people have been greatly helped by this medication. Of course, like all medicines, L-Dopa may have side effects in some people. It must be used cautiously in people with heart disease because it can aggravate cardiac problems. It can also lead to spasms and rigidity on its own. So your doctor will start with a small dose and build it up slowly while watching you carefully.

Not everyone requires L-Dopa. People with milder symptoms may get relief from some of the older medications such as Artane and Cogentin. These drugs block the action of another chemical in the brain (acetylcholine). With less acetylcholine activity, the brain can use whatever dopamine it has more effectively.

Along with medication, physiotherapy is very important. A variety of simple exercises can help keep your muscles limber. Squeezing a small rubber ball, for example, is excellent for the hand and wrist muscles. Rhythmic bending movement at the shoulders, elbows, hips, and knees is also important.

SUMMARY

1. Most elderly people do not suffer significant changes in intellectual capacity although their memory for recent events and quickness of response may be impaired.

2. Many elderly people, particularly those with few hobbies and interests, may suffer from depression and anxiety.

3. If there is a marked change in behavior, the doctor must distinguish between real mental deterioration and psychological problems. He then must ascertain the causes of the problem.

4. In many cases, an elderly person may be suffering from a combination of gradual loss of mental acuity, depression, and anxiety. Each of these problems must be dealt with in an orderly and supportive way in order to help the individual realize his potential for a useful life. This often requires the help of family, friends, doctor, social worker, and counselor.

18

YOUR EYES—
DON'T OVERLOOK THEM

The fabric of our conscious lives is woven of sights and sounds. To all of us, life in a still black night is a chilling thought. It means sensory entombment. But few of us have ever given thought to what life would be like only partially deprived of these senses, living in the twilight world of dimmed sights and muted sounds. Older people with failing vision and hearing frequently encounter this frustrating form of partial isolation. What makes it worse is the failure of friends or relatives to fully appreciate the desperation of someone denied full participation in daily social contacts. For the older person the plight is much worse. Most people will not make allowances for minor inconveniences so that older people can take a part in conversation and social interchange. They find it annoying to have to repeat themselves or extend themselves to make up for someone's impaired perception of the ordinary clues that are so much a part of the normal interaction between people.

But there is something that has an even worse effect on the lives of older people. Too often others fail to recognize that the senses are failing. Even the afflicted person may not be aware of this. It's easy to see how missed or poorly understood words or phrases or mistaken identities can lead to senseless or inappropriate replies. Under these circumstances, an unthinking reaction is to label someone "peculiar" or "odd!" But the older person experiences a far greater humiliation. He's labeled "senile." Friends and relatives shy away rather than be bothered. Slowly the person becomes isolated from his surroundings and is finally totally rejected by those he depends upon for companionship, affection, and support.

In this chapter and the next, we'll take a look at how the eye and ear work and some of the problems likely to develop as we grow older.

THE EYE

Even though the eye is a marvel of complexity, we can understand how it works if we think of it as a camera. The eye itself is a ball, kept inflated by a thick, jellylike fluid. Light enters through the clear window in the front, called the *cornea*. The eye is separated into two compartments by a partition called the *iris*, the colored part of your eye. Light passes through this partition to the back of the eye through the *pupil*, which is simply a hole in the iris. It appears black

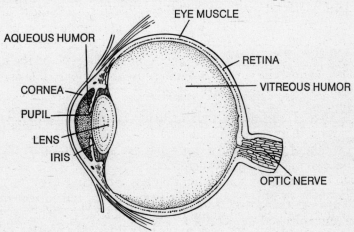

Fig. 29   Normal eye. Light enters the pupil and is focused by the lens on the retina.

because there is no illumination in the back of the eye. By varying its size, the pupil allows just the right amount of light to enter the eye. This is why your pupil becomes smaller in bright light and larger in the dark. Suspended just behind the pupil is a disc-shaped structure called the *lens*. Like the lens of a camera, it focuses the image on the back of the eye, called the *retina*. The image our brain receives is based upon the light messages imprinted on the millions of tiny nerve ends of the retina.

EYELIDS

Each time we blink, we lubricate the delicate surface of our eyes. Our eyelids are also the sole means of protection for the front of our eyes. We blink involuntarily at the slightest threat to our eyes. As the years go by, the tissues of the eyelid weaken and become flabby, just as our skin, often leaving those telltale wrinkles that measure our years like the rings on a tree trunk. As the eyelid loses support, it may seem to shrivel and coil inward or wilt and droop outward. In most cases, the lower lid is affected. As the lid turns inward, the eyelashes begin to brush against the delicate cornea and cause annoying discomfort with tearing and pain. If the lid wilts outward the eye acquires a soulful, dew-eyed expression. This can reduce the lubricating effect of the eye and also lead to irritation and discomfort. Neither condition should be ignored, although the inward coil of the eyelash against the cornea is apt to cause more noticeable symptoms. Often a small strip of adhesive will support the sagging lid, but if the irritation becomes too bothersome, a simple operation should eliminate the problem in either case.

DRY EYES

Tears seem to spring from deep within us under the pressure of uncontrolled emotional forces, much as a geyser erupts under the powerful physical forces that well deep within the earth. The fact is, however, that tears actually come from a number of glands located near the eye.

Many tiny tear glands are scattered throughout the inner surface of our eyelids and provide continuous fine lubrication as we blink. Two larger tear glands lying near the eyeball discharge the more profuse watery tears so obvious to us at times of intense emotion. Tears have a very basic, vital function. Like a sea-living organism, the clear window of our eye, the cornea, requires an aquatic environment. Tears provide this. If you doubt this, try keeping your eyes open for a few minutes without blinking. As soon as the tears dry, you will experience a painful burning sensation. Sometimes the *lacrimal glands*, as the tear glands are called, are unable to make enough fluid to keep the cornea properly lubricated. This condition is referred to as *conjunctivitis sicca*, or simply "dry eyes." The glands that produce saliva may also be afflicted by this form of internal drought, leading to the combination of parched mouth and dry eyes. With fewer tears to bathe them, our eyes begin to sting and burn. Bright lights add to the discomfort. Most of the time, these symptoms are attributed to allergies, irritants in the air, or minor inflammation. As the multiple tiny lubricating glands of the eyelids begin to dry up, the larger tear glands with their greater reserve may release greater quantities of thin, watery tears to compensate. This explains why some people suffering from dry eyes may complain paradoxically that their eyes are always "wet." "Dry eyes" is a relatively minor condition in itself, but neglected for a long time, it can lead to injury of the delicate cornea. Sometimes dry eyes may be part of a more general medical problem. Treatment with eye drops that substitute as tears will prevent drying of the cornea and eliminate the eye irritation.

CATARACTS

After light enters the eye and passes through the pupil, it is focused on the retina by the lens, a small, clear, rubbery, disc-shaped structure lying just behind the pupil. The lens is suspended on mooring lines circumferentially somewhat like a trampoline hung vertically. It is as clear as a fine camera lens and serves a similar purpose. Because of its rubbery character, it can be stretched from a globular to a more

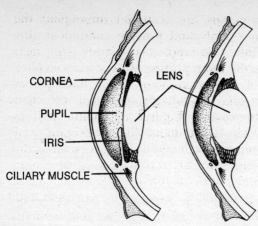

CORNEA

LENS

PUPIL

IRIS

CILIARY MUSCLE

Fig. 30   Elongated normal lens.   Fig. 31   Globular normal lens.
The elasticity of the lens allows it to change shape for focusing.
It is stretched to a more elongated form by contraction of the
ciliary muscles.

elongated shape. This permits us to focus over an infinite
range from very close objects to objects at a great distance.
As you grow older, your lens begins to lose some of its perfect
clarity as well as its rubbery nature. The slight increase in
rigidity may actually improve focusing over a narrower
range. This accounts for the paradox of "renewed vision"
that some older people commonly discover, permitting them
to read without glasses. To most people's dismay, this does
not signal the start of a rejuvenation process. In fact, the
benefits are deceiving. Near vision improves at the expense
of vision for distant objects and the ability to accommodate
for intermediate fields of vision usually suffers. The lens has
simply become stiffer and is less easily stretched. On the
other hand, it is a common experience for many middle-aged
and older people with previous excellent vision to suddenly
find that they require reading glasses. This is an expected
part of growing older and is attributed not to a problem in the
lens itself but to a weakening of the muscle that controls the
shape of the lens.

As the lens becomes somewhat stiff with age, it simultaneously begins to lose some of its transparency although
this may not be obvious. Like drifting clouds, a haziness
slowly, imperceptibly begins to tarnish the lens and eclipse

vision. When this clouding of the lens is visible to a doctor, it is called a *cataract*. Fortunately, most people will never reach this stage or even be aware of any dimming of their vision.

Eye specialists often classify cataracts according to the part of the lens where the clouding process begins. This is not important. What is important is the dimming of vision that results from the cataract. You may have heard of the term "maturity" or "ripeness" of a cataract. This term is meant to indicate that the lens has become milky, turbid, and no longer allows light to pass. Formerly it was believed that before a cataract could be removed it had to reach a state of maturity. This is no longer true and it is now possible to remove any lens that clouds vision. The outer coat of the siliconelike lens may actually liquefy. When this occurs, it is called *hyper-mature* and represents the most serious form of cataract. As it swells it encroaches on adjacent structures in the eye. Protein material leaking from the lens into the eye chamber may cause inflammation of the eye and glaucoma. At this advanced stage, surgery becomes necessary.

Treatment of Cataracts

Most people are surprised when they are told they have cataracts. Their vision seems perfectly normal to them. This is a common situation. The slight clouding of the lens, while evident to the doctor, may no more interfere with vision than a smudge on your eyeglasses. This is usually the extent to which most cataracts progress. So you can rest easy if that is your only problem.

However, when a cataract does interfere with vision, there is no way to dissolve the murkiness in the lens or reverse the clouding process. All that can be done is to remove the cloudy lens. There are several ways to do this. Each can be accomplished simply and easily. Of course without a lens, your vision will be as blurry as a picture taken with a camera without a lens. However, many substitutes are available. For most people, eyeglasses will do nicely. Others might prefer contact lenses if they can be properly fitted. A recent experimental technique involves the insertion of a miniature lens within the eye to replace the extracted lens. Although performed with increasing frequency, this is obviously a more technically demanding procedure, with much greater chance of failure and not suitable for everyone. Patients with other eye problems, such as glaucoma or diabetic retinopathy, are not suited for this type of surgery.

When should cataracts be removed? The answer to this question has changed from time to time. Previously, most specialists thought it wise to wait until the cataract had "matured," that is, had become completely milky before removing it. It is now possible to remove the lens at a much earlier stage. However, a number of factors should be taken into account before deciding on surgery:

1. A cataract takes time to evolve from mild clouding until dense enough to limit vision. If you don't require very fine vision in your daily routines, you can probably wait until the cloudiness becomes an actual hindrance. On the other hand, if you delight in extensive reading or fine handiwork such as needlework, you might not want to wait so long.

2. While cataracts usually occur in both eyes, they may develop at different rates. If only one eye has a cataract, it might be advisable to put off surgery indefinitely. The reason for this is simple. After the lens is removed in only one eye, the special spectacles that must be worn makes it impossible to see with both eyes at the same time. Therefore, you'll still have only one good eye. However, if you are willing to wear a contact lens, this can be fitted on the operated eye. The use of the contact lens permits normal vision with both eyes.

People frequently ask whether it is possible to remove cataracts in both eyes during the same hospital stay. Although this was considered inadvisable in the past, it is current practice now to remove both cataracts during the same week in the hospital. In the five to seven days between removal of the first and second cataract, temporary spectacles will provide satisfactory vision. Both cataracts are never removed at the same time.

3. There are no hard and fast rules about when to have

surgery. One authority suggests that the best time for surgery is when vision is badly impaired in one eye, and the better eye shows signs of deteriorating vision. In the final analysis, the individual, in cooperation with an eye specialist, should make the decision about whether surgery is necessary.

GLAUCOMA

The eye is a fluid-filled ball. It is firmly lodged in the eye socket and constantly acted upon by many powerful muscles that permit you to turn your eyes in many directions (see Fig. 29). A constant pressure is maintained within the eye by a specialized fluid system that keeps the eye ball from collapsing under the strain of many opposing muscles. In the condition called glaucoma, a disturbance in this delicate internal plumbing system leads to a rise of pressure within the eye. To understand how this occurs we need to know something about the normal workings of this internal fluid system.

Two fluid systems support the eye. The larger chamber behind the iris (see page 270) is filled with a thick, jellylike material that occupies most of the eye called the *vitreous humor* (see Fig. 29). The smaller chamber in front is filled with a watery clear fluid called *aqueous humor*. It is the dynamic flow of this latter fluid that controls the pressure within the eye. The fluid is pumped into the eye from behind the iris and flows to the front of the eye where it drains out of the eye. Pressure remains constant as long as the amount draining equals the amount of fluid entering, much as the pressure behind a dam remains constant as long as its outflow balances its inflow. Pressure will rise if the drainage system becomes clogged and fluid continues to pour in. This is precisely what happens in glaucoma. While the reasons for the clogged runoff may vary, the final result is the same: rising pressure within the eye.

Symptoms of Glaucoma

It is not without reason that glaucoma is called the sneak thief of sight. In the more common type, called *chronic sim-*

ple glaucoma or *open angle type*, pressure rises slowly and often fluctuates, and symptoms progress insidiously.

An entirely different situation exists when the pressure in the eye rises suddenly. This is the case in the condition called *closed angle* or *acute glaucoma*. The attack appears explosively with severe pain, nausea, and vomiting. A thick fog rolls across the field of vision. Ordinary light becomes a searing flash. The pain resembles a gripping headache and it may not be apparent at first that the problem is coming from the eye. This represents a true emergency and an eye specialist must be consulted at once.

Another less common type of glaucoma behaves less dramatically. In this type, pain is often less intense and a rainbow halo intermittently seems to surround streetlights. Never neglect any symptom no matter how subtle. Certain people are at a higher risk for glaucoma and should be particularly vigilant to any change in vision. This includes those with a family history of glaucoma or diabetes. A yearly checkup is wise in such cases.

Why all the concern about a rising pressure within the eye? The answer is obvious. When the pressure rises, something must give. Since the eyeball itself is composed of a tough sheath, there is no chance of an explosive blowout as in an overinflated tire. Rather, rising pressure seeks release by compressing the jellylike fluid in the back of the eye forcing it against the delicate and vital retinal lining of the eye. Eventually, injury to these nerves will result in a gradual loss of vision, and, if untreated, blindness.

Diagnosis and Treatment of Glaucoma

There is only one sure way to diagnose glaucoma. This is to measure the pressure in the eyeball. Remember, the best time to diagnose the condition is before trouble begins. Often your doctor can judge whether a problem exists by simply inspecting the back of your eye. To be absolutely certain, however, it is necessary to directly measure the pressure in the eye. This is a simple procedure and takes only a few minutes. It is just a matter of putting a few drops into your eyes and placing a small instrument directly against the eye. A casual visit to your optometrist for checkup of your eyeglasses is no substitute for a thorough, proper examination. As we have seen, glaucoma is not one disease, but a series of conditions having one thing in common, elevated pressure in the eye. When the pressure is elevated without any evidence of injury to the eye, specialists sometimes use the term *ocular hypertension* or *glaucoma suspect*. In such cases they may choose not to treat immediately but to follow with frequent eye examinations.

For most people, the treatment of glaucoma involves nothing more than putting a few drops into the eye each day. One type of eye drop that is used will cause the pupil to become smaller. You may notice that it is difficult to accommodate to the dark, since the pupil is unable to open wide. The most commonly used medication of this type is called pilocarpine. Other types of drugs may have hardly any effect on the pupil. Epinephrine is one. Timolol is a newer drug that does not affect the pupil at all. Never use more than the prescribed amount because they can be absorbed into your body and cause side effects.

On occasion it may be necessary to reduce the fluid production using a pill called Diamox (acetozolamide). In reality this is a type of diuretic, or water pill.

It is necessary to act more quickly with the explosive attack of closed angle glaucoma since sight is immediately threatened. This is accomplished first by the use of eyedrops. If this fails to relieve the condition, Diamox may be given by injection. In severe cases medication may be given by vein to draw fluid from the eye and relieve the pressure, or a sweet-tasting solution can be taken by mouth called glycerol, which accomplishes the same purpose.

Surgery is usually required to prevent future attacks in the closed angle type of glaucoma. Eye drops will usually suffice in the most common open angle type. Nevertheless, even here, close supervision is necessary to insure that the pressure remains normal. Surgery should be considered only when medicines fail. The eye specialist can monitor the effectiveness of treatment by measuring pressure periodically. In addition, he will watch over the condition of the eye by examining the nerve in back of the eye and evaluating

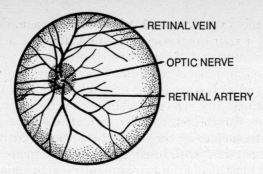

RETINAL VEIN

OPTIC NERVE

RETINAL ARTERY

Fig. 32 View of the retina as seen by the doctor through an ophthalmoscope.

vision by the simple test called *visual fields*. One of the situations where removal of cataracts seems advisable occurs
when cataracts and glaucoma coexist. Cataracts may make
it impossible to properly examine the back of the eye for
signs of injury to the eye from glaucoma.

RETINAL PROBLEMS

The retina, or the lining of the back of the eye, is a living
photographic plate (see Fig. 29). Here all the images that
enter the eye are recorded and transmitted to the brain. It is
the command post, regulating the entire complex function of
the eye, the vital center of sight. In addition, it is the only
part of the body where living blood vessels can be seen directly, a window to the living circulation. When your doctor
peers into your eyes with the light from an *ophthalmoscope*,
he sees the central area where the main transmission cable
of sight, the *optic nerve*, leaves the eye, and, in addition, the
vinelike blood vessels reaching out to the back of the eye in
many directions. Many of the most dramatic scenes of medical illness acting on the whole body are played out on this
retinal stage. Specific signs remain that can be deciphered by
your doctor. Diseases that affect the blood vessels of the
body may be clearly evaluated by the effect they have on the
blood vessels of the eye. Diabetes and high blood pressure
are two common examples of the type of conditions that can
be analyzed by examining the retina.

It is obvious that this delicate lining is susceptible to injury by a variety of conditions. We shall touch on only two of these, diabetes and retinal detachment.

Diabetic Retinopathy

Diabetes seems to deal unfairly with the eye. Cataracts and glaucoma occur more commonly in diabetes. But it is damage to the retina that represents the major threat to vision. The blood vessels of the eye are often the first to show the impact diabetes has on the blood vessels of the body. It is here that the doctor may actually first discover the telltale signs of diabetes, the *microaneurysm*, a tiny red dot, signifying a bulge in the wall of a blood vessel. By themselves, these changes don't cause any problem. But leakage of blood from these tiny blood vessels can lead to injury particularly when repeated bouts of seepage result in scarring. Tiny new blood vessels may invade the scars and the jellylike fluid in the back of the eye (vitreous humor). Ultimately, this can threaten vision.

People with diabetes should have periodic eye examinations. Not only can the condition of the eyes be closely followed, but in certain instances it is possible to arrest the damaging effect of a leaking vessel, using laser instruments to cauterize these areas. Tiny leaks can be detected by injecting a special dye called *fluorescein* into a vein and observing its escape through blood vessels in the eye. In addition, laser therapy has been shown to significantly reduce major loss of vision in cases of growth of blood vessels into the vitreous. While not everyone agrees on the total effectiveness of the new form of therapy or the exact time to initiate it, it will continue to play an increasing role in the management of the problem.

A more radical type of treatment involves removal of this entire thick jelly and substituting an artificial fluid. This is attempted only when bleeding into the vitreous has led to severe diminution of vision. Clearly this has much higher risks and is applicable only to few people.

If you have diabetes, don't panic. Few people ever develop serious injury to the blood vessels in their eyes. Fewer

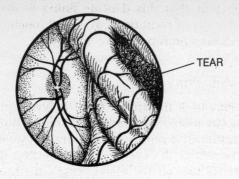

TEAR

Fig. 33   Retinal detachment. If the retina is torn in any area, it begins to lift up from the back of the eye.

still stand the risk of losing vision. Nevertheless, it makes good sense to have a periodic eye examination. If a problem does occur, it may be caught early and treated.

Retinal Detachment

The retinal lining is firmly attached to the underlying layer of the eye, but like the rind of an orange it can be separated from this layer. In so doing it is uprooted from the blood supply that nourishes it and suffers serious injury. This is what is referred to as retinal detachment. It represents a serious condition particularly since the retina may continue to peel from its base, isolating it from its nutritional source.

While the retina may detach suddenly, more often than not there will be some warning. Commonly, floating spots will suddenly appear in one eye. This must not be mistaken for the common "floaters" that just about everyone experiences at one time or another. These harmless floaters seem to swim across our field of vision and disappear like delicate, diaphanous sea creatures. Often we can summon their return with a quick turn of our eyes. They represent some cells from inside the eye and will settle from our view unless we churn them up. The spots from a retinal detachment are an entirely different matter. They are smaller and more numerous flashes of light, like a snow flurry, and can't be ignored because they interfere with vision. Unlike harmless black floaters that briefly blow across our vision, the disturbances of a retinal detachment persist. They represent slight seepage of blood from a tear in the retina that precedes the actual separation of the retina. Although you may breathe a sigh of relief when these spots finally fade after a day or so, it is anything but a good omen. The blood particles that have caused the disturbance will settle out and vision will return to normal. But the stage has been set for the more serious events to follow as the retina prepares to work itself loose and slowly peel from the underlying wall.

Don't let this quiescent phase lull you into inaction if you haven't sought help when the spots first appeared. The real danger is about to begin. As the retina is lifted off, vision is slowly lost. Usually this begins in the periphery of the eye and slowly approaches the center. The condition is painless, and since the usual loss of vision is at the extreme corner of vision, many people actually ignore the condition or may remain totally unaware of it at first. If a large section tears loose, vision may be abruptly eclipsed. This is often described as a curtain being pulled across the field of vision. An uncommon but treacherous situation may develop as sight temporarily improves overnight as the retinal layer drops back to its base, aided by the force of gravity. This can lull you into a false sense of security, since it is easy to convince yourself that things are improving. Don't take chances. Seek help immediately before lasting damage is done.

The treatment of retinal detachment is relatively straightforward. Tiny areas of inflammation are provoked in the layer beneath the retina, which will grip the loose retinal lining and firmly bond it. Diathermy was previously used but recently cryotherapy (treatment by freezing) has proved to be remarkably effective. In less than a week most patients are out of the hospital. The reattachment of the retina is quite permanent. Less than one in ten people experience a new detachment. If caught early enough, laser therapy can be used to seal holes in the retina before actual detachment occurs.

SUMMARY

1. Cataracts are nothing more than a fogging of the lens of the eye. If your eyesight is good, don't panic if you are told you have cataracts. On the other hand, if your vision is poor because of cataracts, they can be easily removed and replaced by a substitute lens.

2. Glaucoma is one of the leading causes of blindness. Yet it is treatable and if caught early, loss of vision can be prevented. But the best way to be certain is to have the pressure in your eyes checked at least every year.

3. If you are a diabetic, be sure to have an eye examination at regular intervals—at least once a year.

4. Remember, any unusual visual disturbance, such as persistent spots or missing slices of vision, may be early warnings of a retinal detachment. Don't be misled by the absence of pain or a slight improvement. See your eye doctor immediately.

19

YOUR EARS—
GIVE THEM A FAIR HEARING

Minor loss of hearing is usually considered more of a nuisance than a real handicap. It is often dismissed as an inevitable consequence of growing older. We generally first have difficulty hearing higher tones. This makes it easier to accept. What's the difference if ringing bells seem muffled or we miss the treetop melodies of a spring day? And how many of us listen for the solitary flute in a symphony anyway? But such logic misses the point. We are awash in sounds at every turn. They guide us, warn us, bind us to others. From the shrill warning of a honking horn to the faint voice behind us trying to attract our attention, we rely on sound in so many ways. Language is the currency of human exchange. The word-to-word link that forms the chain of conversation binds us to one another. A lost word is a broken link in this chain.

Hearing loss may come on gradually as hearing fades almost imperceptibly. At first whispers become faint mumbles. Speakers seem farther away than they really are. Later, words of normal conversation seem to ebb and flow like a weak transmission from a distant radio station. The person can no longer participate fully as he loses words or phrases.

284

Even patient friends and relatives tire at having to repeat themselves or shout to make themselves understood. Dispirited, the person voluntarily withdraws and becomes more and more the outsider. At times, he may attempt to compensate by guessing at missed segments of conversation. But this usually doesn't last long as inappropriate replies or irrelevant topics interjected in the middle of conversation quickly become annoying to others. The person with a conductive hearing loss (see page 286) finds the sound of his own voice loud and shrill and gradually lowers it to the point of barely being understood.

It doesn't take long before this type of behavior is ascribed to memory or concentration lapses or worse yet, failing intellect. And if you happen to be old when this happens, you're labeled senile. This isn't at all far-fetched. It happens all the time. And there is no need for it. Help is available in the form of compact and comfortable hearing aids.

We'll come back to this, but first, let's look at how the ear normally functions.

HOW WE HEAR

Sound reaches our brain through a complicated relay system. The ear drum, a taut membrane at the end of the ear canal, vibrates at the impact of sound waves, much as the covering of a drum does when struck. This sets in motion a series of three small bones lying just behind the ear drum in a chamber called the *middle ear*. The vibration of these bones sends ripples through a tightly sealed fluid system, locked deep in the bony recesses of our skull, called the *inner ear* or *cochlea*. The movements in this fluid are carried by the auditory nerve to the brain where they are interpreted as sound messages (see page 286). This complex relay system can be interrupted at any point along the way.

Hearing loss is usually divided into two major disruptions in the sound pathway. A hearing problem resulting from damage to the inner ear (cochlea) or auditory nerve

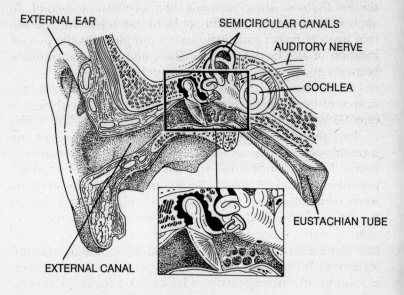

EXTERNAL EAR

SEMICIRCULAR CANALS

AUDITORY NERVE

COCHLEA

EUSTACHIAN TUBE

EXTERNAL CANAL

Fig. 34   Anatomy of the normal ear. Insert shows the middle ear. (See
Fig. 35). The inner ear consists of the semicircular canals,
cochlea, and auditory nerve.

is referred to as *nerve deafness* whereas injury to the middle
ear is said to cause *conduction deafness*. Using a tuning fork,
your doctor can often discriminate between these two types
of hearing loss. When a vibrating tuning fork is held near
your ear, the sound waves must travel through the entire
conducting system, from the ear drum along the bones of the
middle ear finally passing through the cochlea and auditory
nerve. If the vibrating tuning fork is pressed against your
head, sound waves are conducted directly through the skull
bones to the cochlea and auditory nerve, completely bypass-
ing the middle ear. Thus, if hearing loss is due to injury to
the middle ear (conduction disturbance) you can hear the
vibrations when the tuning fork touches your head even

though sound has faded when it is held beside your ear. On the other hand, if there is nerve deafness the vibrations will not be heard no matter where the tuning fork is placed since the final part of the communication system is impaired. In such a case hearing aids will not be of much benefit. Specialized hearing tests (audiologic tests) can pinpoint the precise location of the hearing malfunction and even discriminate between injury to the cochlea or auditory nerve.

It is normal for older people to develop some minor degree of hearing loss for high frequency sound although it may be so minor that only sensitive hearing tests can detect it. This probably involves changes in several areas of the transmission system in the ear, particularly the auditory nerve. These changes are expected and usually have no noticeable effect on hearing. Sometimes there may even be some compensations. Loud and harsh high-pitched sounds are muted and lose their shrill irritation. So, in some ways things balance out for most people. If the changes go beyond this point, however, sound may be muffled enough to cause serious inconvenience. When this happens, a thorough examination by an ear specialist is advisable. Chances are that he will find no definable damage, and a hearing aid is all that will be necessary. Sometimes specific conditions will be to blame. Here are a few of the most common ones.

OTITIS MEDIA

Otitis simply means inflammation of the ear. Since the ear has several compartments, the exact location must be found. Thus if the inflammation involves only the short canal leading to the ear drum, it is referred to as *otitis externa*, while involvement of the small compartment behind the ear drum is *otitis media*.

Infection in the outer canal may result in discomfort, itching, and drainage, which should not cause much concern. But occasionally severe pain may result and in diabetics the condition can be a serious matter. Inflammation of the middle ear chamber is an entirely different condition. Attacks of middle ear infection are quite common in infants and young people, but rarely develop later in life. At any age, pain, fever, and drainage make it difficult to overlook when it does occur. However, the consequence of multiple infections on hearing may not become apparent until a later age. The hearing loss due to otitis media is a conductive type and hearing aids are generally beneficial.

One unusual but potentially serious consequence of long-standing, simmering inflammation in the middle ear is *cholesteatoma,* a cystlike accumulation of whitish silvery debris. As the years go by, it slowly enlarges and encroaches on adjacent structures, eventually eroding them. The condition can be identified by a doctor by a simple examination of the ear. If left unattended, irreparable damage to the middle ear and even worse consequences can ultimately develop. It can usually be eradicated by surgery.

OTOSCLEROSIS

Three tiny bones closely linked to one another lie nestled in the middle ear chamber behind the ear drum. They resemble a miniature hammer, anvil, and stirrup, but perhaps to avoid the unseeming image of a livery stable they are known by the Latin names for these structures. The third bone in series, the *stapes* or *stirrup*, occupies a critical position, since its footplate caps the entrance to the spiral, fluid-filled chamber of the inner ear. Sound waves strike the ear drum setting the three bones of the middle ear in motion, agitating the stapes, which sends gentle ripples through the canal of the inner ear. These rolling waves are the sound messages carried to our brain by the auditory nerve.

In the condition called *otosclerosis*, an overgrowth of bony tissue slowly freezes the free movement of the stapes, dampening its vibration (fig. 36). The stapes occupies a critical position because its delicate piston action must transmit sound directly to the fluid of the inner ear. The condition may begin in adolescence but progresses throughout life. Hearing loss may not be apparent until later in life. Great strides in microsurgical technique have made it possible to remove the diminutive stapes and replace it with an artificial graft, restoring hearing to those once closeted in silence.

MÉNIÈRE'S DISEASE

Locked securely within the bony vault of our skull behind the middle ear is a coiled fluid-filled canal, winding in spiral fashion like a sea shell. This is the *inner ear* or *cochlea* (see p. 285). You might think that hearing and balance should have nothing to do with one another, yet they are intimately related. Our internal gyroscope that allows us to orient ourselves in space is composed of several circular fluid-filled canals (semicircular canals) located in the inner ear. Al-

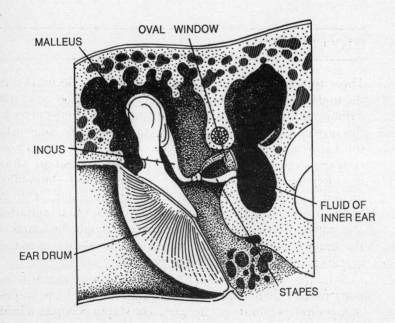

Fig. 35   Close-up of middle ear. Sound waves striking the eardrum set the malleus in motion. This motion is transmitted to the incus and stapes. Note that the stapes caps the entrance to the fluid-filled inner ear (oval window). Agitation of this fluid is ultimately transmitted as sound messages through the auditory nerve.

though the fluid circulates in a closed system, at one point it communicates with the fluid in one of the canals carrying sound vibrations, establishing a direct physical link between balance and hearing.

Usually the first thing that is noticed is ringing in the ears, called *tinnitus*, and loss of hearing. This is followed by explosive attacks of dizziness, some mild, some more severe, which can vary considerably, some lasting up to a few days, but often less than an hour. Surroundings seem to spin, as though the person were perched on a slowly reeling, un-balanced carousel. Severe nausea and vomiting are not un-usual. During the attack and often just preceding it, the ringing may increase in intensity. Mild hearing loss during and after the attack improves, but less so with each succes-sive episode. Because in most cases only one ear is involved, the loss of hearing may not be readily apparent.

The condition seems to be related to a build-up of fluid and pressure within the canals of the inner ear. Since the attacks usually subside within several hours, medicines to control the nausea while you rest in bed are all that is generally required. A drug that seems to be particularly effective is diazepam (Valium), often given with an anti-cholinergic medicine. To reduce the fluid accumulation between attacks, a low salt diet, reduced fluid intake, and a diuretic are helpful. Surgery is considered only when at-tacks are frequent and incapacitating. This involves either total surgical destruction of the balance and hearing mech-anism or selective destruction by beaming high frequency sound waves into the inner ear. The latter approach is more prone to failure, but does preserve hearing when successful.

It is important to realize that not every attack of dizzi-ness or ringing in the ears is due to Ménière's disease. The delicate mechanism of the inner ear is susceptible to many forms of injury. Minor viral infections, allergies, drugs, or even sinus and ear infections can lead to identical symptoms.

A slow growing and treatable tumor called an *acoustic neuroma* can be easily mistaken for Ménière's disease. The fact that both conditions are less often seen in older people could lead to needless delay if the possibility of a tumor is not immediately considered.

A stroke may begin with dizziness and nausea, but other signs usually assist the doctor in ruling out this problem.

Nevertheless, the diagnosis of a sudden attack of dizziness is not always easy. So if your doctor decides he needs more tests before he is satisfied about the diagnosis, bear with him.

DRUGS AND THE EAR

In many areas, medical progress involves a tradeoff—we risk some harm for the greater good. This is particularly so with medicines. Unlike the liver, the ear is generally spared the brunt of side effects of drugs. Still, certain medications can

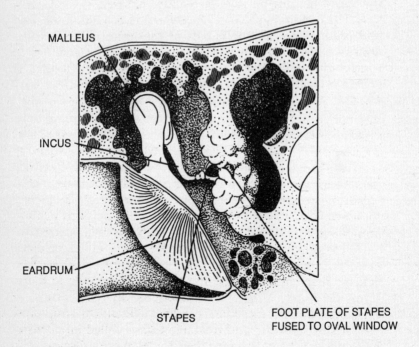

Fig. 36   Middle ear in otosclerosis. Note that the footplate of the stapes is fused by bony overgrowth to the entrance of the inner ear (oval window).

injure the ear and affect hearing or balance. Certain antibiotics, often used for life-threatening infections, can cause
problems here. The same is true for water pills used in huge
quantities in people with serious kidney ailments. Aspirin,
when used in large quantities, can cause ringing in the ears,
as can indomethacin, quinidine, and chlorpromazine. Because aspirin is used so commonly, it is often not even regarded as medicine, but you should mention it to your doctor
if you take aspirin.

RINGING IN THE EARS

Ringing in the ears barely seems worth talking about. It
usually passes quickly and is merely an annoyance. We expect it after such sudden loud sounds as a firecracker. Sometimes, however, the ringing doesn't fade away. It can have
many qualities, from the loud, high-pitched tone so irritating
with the test pattern on a TV station to the low rumble of a
sea surf. Older people may be reluctant even to mention this
problem even when the ringing persists. When it is mentioned, the glances in reply seem to say, "Now he's hearing
things." This is unfortunate since ringing in the ear can
cause considerable discomfort and upset one's life.

Most of the time it is caused by a minor problem, such as
ear wax, sinus, or ear infection or a clogged Eustachean tube
(see fig. 34). The latter is a small passage from the back
of the throat to the middle ear chamber that keeps the pressure equal on both sides of the ear drum. You open it when
you swallow to unclog your ears after changing altitudes as
in an airplane or elevator. Even unsuspected dental conditions or arthritis of the jaw can lead to ringing in the ears.
Certain drugs may also be responsible (see above). Still,
since more serious conditions such as tumors or Ménière's
disease (see page 289) can also result in ringing in the ears,
always have a checkup if the ringing fails to disappear.

Most often doctors find no cause and people must learn
to live with the monotonous hum. Some highly imaginative
approaches have been tried for those people who are driven

to distraction by the interminable ringing, including sub-stituting a more acceptable tone to mask the unpleasant ringing. This is accomplished by a small transmitting device worn much the way a hearing aid is.

SUMMARY

1. Hearing is too often taken for granted. If hearing loss is not recognized, serious disruption of normal life can occur. Even worse, it can lead to being ostracized as senile, the modern equivalent of leprosy.

2. Modern hearing aids have restored even severely impaired hearing.

3. Hearing and balance are often related and problems with both may indicate a disturbance of the inner ear.

4. Ringing in the ears is a common problem. Still, a complete checkup is in order if this persists. Only rarely will any serious problem be found. Don't be shy about seeking help. That is a real ring you are hearing.

20

CHOOSING
A DOCTOR

In this book we have tried to give you an understanding of
what it means to grow older, to help you distinguish abnormal symptoms from normal changes, and to enable you to
decide when you need professional help. We have also
pointed out a few areas where you should have regular
checkups.

We are assuming, of course, that you have a congenial
and competent family physician who will minister not only
to your physical ills but also to your emotional problems and
fears. We know, however, that it isn't easy to find this kind
of doctor. It never has been. Nevertheless you can't escape
the responsibility for finding and choosing the doctor who
will be best for you.

PERSONAL QUALITIES OF A DOCTOR

Before you choose a doctor, think about the kind of person
you would like him or her to be. You should be looking for
such qualities as a sense of humor, an ability to make you
feel secure, speech and manner that inspire confidence. You
want someone you can talk with frankly and fully. You want

your doctor to understand you and to treat you effectively and sympathetically.

It's a tall order, but anything less isn't good enough. We can't help you choose the doctor who makes you feel good, likes you, treats you warmly, humanly. Only you can tell whether your doctor has these qualities. He may have them for you, but others may feel quite different about him. It's the same here as in every other personal relationship. It's based on purely subjective feelings—very important, but still subjective. And, in a very real sense, not always the most important characteristics of the good physician.

Too many people choose their doctors primarily for certain superficial likeability, cheerfulness, hail-fellow-well-met qualities. Others are impressed with the affable, reassuring father figure. We would not in any way underrate these qualities in a physician. But, underneath these very attractive traits, there must be some substance, some solid knowledge, training, judgment, and experience. After all, these are what count most. They determine, in large measure, whether the doctor understands what is bothering you and what he has to do to relieve your distress. Personal charm, kindliness, fatherliness, and compassion are no substitutes for knowledge and experience, and the ability to apply it.

THE IDEAL DOCTOR

What is the ideal family physician like? First, he is compulsive about details. He wants to understand your symptoms in great detail. To do this, he must be willing to spend time with you, listen attentively, and then examine you carefully and thoroughly. The practitioner who waltzes thirty patients through his office in a few hours cannot possibly do his job adequately. Over the long haul, he is bound to miss some important findings. Your health is too precious to trust to this kind of high-volume doctor.

Your doctor should be extremely conscientious, and being extremely conscientious does not mean ordering a multitude of laboratory tests for every symptom. This is not sound judgment. He should do a thorough follow-up of every significant complaint but avoid unnecessary tests. Certain tests—such as Pap smears for women, examination of stool for blood, and mammography for certain women at high risk for breast cancer—he should order on a regular basis.

KNOWLEDGE AND JUDGMENT

Look for good medical judgment in your doctor. This judgment is based on two elements: medical knowledge and the ability to use it. Thus, your doctor must be well educated not only in book knowledge but in that kind of knowledge that comes only with experience and is tempered by good common sense. The doctor you want must know when a problem is trivial, when it requires further investigation, when it is urgent, and when it is not. Most important, he must know when he needs help. He does not have to be a genius nor does he have to know everything about every illness. But he must know when to call in a consultant, someone who knows more than he does about a particular problem. With common sense, experience, and humility, your doctor is likely to do a good job. Without these qualities, he will make dreadful errors no matter how many facts he has memorized.

Your doctor should remain a student in his profession. Our concepts about so many diseases, including diagnosis and treatment, change rapidly. New information appears almost daily. A good doctor must keep up with all these new concepts if he is to treat you well. Your doctor may finish his formal training knowing a great deal. But he will be out of date within a few years if he doesn't read medical journals and attend lectures, meetings, and demonstrations.

HOW TO FIND A GOOD DOCTOR

How do you go about finding this conscientious, careful, informed, competent doctor? Frankly, it's not easy for the layman to make this kind of choice. After all, it's always difficult to judge the competence and reliability of anyone who is doing something we know very little about. This is true whether we are choosing a plumber, electrician, lawyer, or doctor. Choosing a doctor is especially difficult. Here you're not dealing with something like a cabinet, for example, where you can see the carpenter's craftsmanship, the quality of design, wood, and finish. You can, on the basis of what you see, decide whether you want the carpenter to create something for you, or to provide you with other similar services or products.

It isn't so easy, however, to judge the quality of a doctor's services. Even his fellow doctors frequently have some difficulty in judging his competence. The obvious differences between a good doctor and a mediocre or poor one are often very small indeed. Most patients will recover no matter what the doctor does. A few will not get better despite their doctor's best efforts. For a relatively small number of people, what the doctor does or does not do makes a real difference. Thus, you can't judge a doctor entirely by the few people who have recovered under his care, or by the few very sick people who did not improve. Before you could make a really valid judgment, you would have to observe how your doctor functions in many situations with various kinds of patients. This is obviously something you aren't prepared to do. The reactions and recommendations of your friends and relatives aren't always too reliable either, although this is how a great many people choose their doctors.

Where does this leave you now? Your feelings about your doctor don't really tell you how good a doctor he is. Your friends and relatives aren't wholly reliable judges either. What else can you do to make reasonably certain that your doctor is a well-trained, well-qualified, decent, kind human being?

Here are some important things you should do and consider, some questions you should get answers to. They should help you find the doctor who is right for you.

First, look for a family doctor who can handle 90 percent of the problems he runs into and who knows when to send you to a specialist for a complex problem he doesn't feel he can deal with. Part of being a good doctor is knowing when to refer your patient to someone with more specialized expertise. You do not want to go to a gastroenterologist every time you feel nauseated or to a cardiologist every time you have a pain in your chest. So start your search for a family doctor by limiting yourself to someone who has had training in internal medicine or family practice. In both cases, the doctor will have had to spend at least three years beyond medical school practicing in a hospital where he has encountered a wide variety of illnesses, and where he has been supervised and taught by an experienced group of well-trained doctors.

Such groups as the American Medical Association and the American Boards of Internal Medicine and Family Practice must approve these training programs. At the end of the training period, each doctor takes an examination and if he passes it, becomes board certified in internal medicine or family practice. You can look for the doctor's name in the *Directory of Medical Specialists*, which is available in libraries or at your state or local Medical Society. If he is board certified, you have already found one measure of his competence.

One good way to find a family doctor is to call a good voluntary (nonprofit) hospital and ask for a list of recommended physicians in your neighborhood. Then choose one who is board certified. In order to narrow the choice even further, look up the names of the hospitals where he has trained. Generally, those hospitals intimately connected with a medical school provide excellent training. The directory will also tell you whether your doctor has a faculty appointment at a medical school. This appointment is often quite significant. It usually means that he spends some time teaching students and training other doctors. To do this, he must have a real interest in what is happening in the field of medicine. He must be interested, too, in teaching others what he knows. And very important, he must have been judged highly competent as a teacher by the medical school officials.

After you have chosen a doctor, call his office for an appointment. Unless you are in some kind of emergency situation, allow for a reasonable waiting period. But if you have to wait weeks to see the doctor, seriously consider choosing another doctor. A doctor's qualifications, credentials, reputation, and recommendations aren't much use to you if you can't get to see him when you need him.

THE FIRST VISIT

When you go to the physician's office for the first time, observe him carefully. Does he run from one patient examining room to another? Is he a good listener? Does he ask detailed questions? Does he answer all your questions fully and simply? Is he thorough in his examination, starting from your head and working down to your feet? Does he do a careful physical examination? (See checklist, page 300).

After the examination is complete, does your doctor explain what he has found, what further tests he wants you to take and why he has ordered each test and medication? Does he make it easy for you to ask detailed questions? In short, does he leave you with a good understanding of what he is doing and why he is doing it? It is very important to have a physician who is willing to discuss your problems with you. Unfortunately, we find that most patients know very little about their medical problems and are taking many important medicines without any real understanding of what they are supposed to do for them. They rarely know anything about the side effects of these drugs or the danger signs to watch for. If their doctors had taken the time and trouble to discuss their medicines with them, many people could avoid serious reactions by recognizing their warning signs, stopping the medicine, and calling their doctor.

It is also very important to have a physician who is willing to share the burden of major decisions with others. You should not be afraid to ask for a second opinion if you are insecure about the advice you receive. A secure, reliable physician should be willing to refer you to a competent specialist for the second opinion.

Doctors are often notoriously negligent in discussing diets and nutrition with their patients. Telling you to stay on a low-salt or low-fat diet is not very helpful unless you know why. You need to know exactly what you can eat and what you can't eat. Doctors who don't give this information to their patients aren't fully meeting their responsibilities. Diet plays an important role in such conditions as diabetes and heart disease, for example. A doctor's failure to make this information available to his patients amounts almost to neglect of professional duty, especially when this information is so easily available at no expense to doctor or patient.

On your first visit, find out how comprehensive your physician's services are. Is there medical coverage for his patients twenty-four hours a day? Is night coverage handled by inexperienced residents or by other experienced physicians? There are some excellent group practices and partnerships that insure the availability of a well-trained physician at all times.

You should know what hospitals your doctor uses for his patients. By and large, voluntary hospitals are the best, particularly those with internists in training on duty at all times. You should generally stay away from physicians who use only proprietary hospitals (privately owned and run as profit-making businesses). They may lack the ability to obtain privileges at a major hospital or are not willing or able to shoulder the load of teaching and clinical work required of all doctors who may admit patients to these hospitals.

Choosing a physician carefully is a difficult but important job. But you won't get the medical care you deserve unless you choose your doctor carefully. If you have found a careful, competent, compassionate physician who takes the time to talk to you, hold on to him. You have a real gem.

WHAT YOUR DOCTOR SHOULD CHECK AT LEAST ONCE A YEAR

1. Check vital signs—blood pressure in both arms, pulse rate, and temperature
2. Look with light in ears, throat, and eyes
3. Look inside eyes with bright light in a dark room
4. Check eye movements and tongue movements

5. Palpate along sides of neck for lymph nodes
6. Palpate thyroid gland in front part of neck
7. Check neck movements
8. Take some time in carefully examining the chest, listening in several different areas
9. Palpate the heartbeat on the left side of the chest
10. Listen to the heart with the stethoscope in four or five places on the chest
11. Palpate entire abdomen while patient is lying comfortably on his back
12. Listen to the abdomen with the stethoscope
13. Check the pulses in the groin, under the knee, at the ankle and on the foot
14. Check strength of arms and legs and movements of face
15. Check the reflexes at the knees, ankles, and elbows
16. Check sensation in the arms and legs
17. In men, rectal examination and palpation of testicles
18. In women, careful palpation of breasts, vaginal examination, and rectal examination

21

SOME COMMON MEDICINES:
HOW THEY HELP
AND HARM

(* denotes brand name; all others, generic names)

ACETAMINOPHEN (TYLENOL*, DATRIL*)
Effect:
1) Pain reliever like aspirin, but does not relieve inflammation.
2) Reduces fever.
Side Effect:
High doses can lead to liver damage.

ALDACTONE* (SPIRONOLACTONE)
Effect:
1) Increases loss of water and salt through kidneys.
2) Lowers blood pressure.
Side Effects:
1) Same as chlorothiazide (1).
2) Too much potassium retention leading to abnormal
heart rhythm.
3) Swelling of breasts in males.

ALDOMET* (METHYL DOPA)
Effect:
Lowers blood pressure.
Side Effects:
1) Dizziness on standing up (orthostatic hypotension).
2) Occasional impotence, which disappears rapidly when dosage is stopped.
3) Occasional anemia due to antibodies that destroy red blood cells.
4) Liver injury.
Advice:
May cause you to feel weak and sleepy for the first two weeks, but this effect will generally wear off. Rise slowly to standing position after sitting or lying down.

ALLOPURINOL (ZYLOPRIM*)
Effect:
Prevents uric acid from building up in blood; useful in people with tendency to gout or uric acid kidney stones.
Side Effect:
1) Allergic reactions, skin rashes, and fever.
2) Nausea.
Advice:
This drug should not be taken for several weeks after an episode of gout because it might precipitate another attack.

AMITRIL* (AMITRIPTYLINE) See tricyclic antidepressant drugs.

AMPICILLIN
Effect:
1) A modified penicillin that is effective against most of the bacteria that cause kidney, gall bladder, and gastrointestinal infections.
2) Also useful for patients with emphysema.
Side Effect:
Same as penicillin.
Advice:
If you have an allergic reaction to one kind of penicillin, you are allergic to all the others also.

ANTACIDS
Effect:

Neutralizes acid; used in treatment of peptic ulcer, esophagitis and heartburn.

Side Effects:
1) Diarrhea.
2) Constipation.

ANTICHOLINERGIC DRUGS
Effect:
1) Reduce stomach acid.
2) Slow intestinal motility.

Side Effects:
1) Dry mouth.
2) Blurred vision.
3) Rapid heart rate.
4) Difficulty in urination.
5) Raise pressure in eye in people with glaucoma.
6) Constipation.

Advice:

Must be avoided by people with glaucoma or men with prostate trouble.

ANTIHISTAMINES
Effects:

Blocks action of histamine, a substance produced in excess in allergic persons.

Side Effects:
1) Drowsiness.
2) Dry mouth.
3) Upset stomach.
4) Acne.
5) Reduces healing of wounds.
6) Can lead to cataracts after long-term use.
7) Thins skin and causes easy bruising.

Advice:

Never use without close medical supervision. Never stop suddenly.

ANTURANE (SULFINPYRAZONE)
Effect:

Lowers uric acid level in blood by increasing excretion in urine; reduces clotting by effect on platelets. Used for treatment of gout. Recently used to reduce chances of second heart attack.

Side Effects:
1) Nausea, indigestion, stomach pains.
2) Rash.

Advice:
Should not be used by people with peptic ulcers since it may aggravate ulcers. Should be avoided by people with uric acid kidney stones.

ARTANE* (TRIHEXYPHENIDYL)

Effect:
1) Treatment of rigidity and tremors in Parkinson's disease.
2) Used to control the same type of symptoms in people taking large doses of phenothiazine tranquilizers.

Side Effects:
Same as anticholinergic medicines.

ASPIRIN

Effects:
1) Relieves pain.
2) Relieves inflammation; useful for treatment of arthritis.
3) Acts as an anticoagulant by blocking the action of blood platelets; useful for men in preventing strokes.
4) Reduces fever.

Side Effects:
1) Stomach irritation and ulcer.
2) Bleeding especially from stomach.
3) Ringing in the ears.

Advice:
Take with food or antacid and never on empty stomach. If you take aspirin regularly, watch the color of your stool; if it turns black, check with your physician immediately.

BACTRIM* (TRIMETHOPRIM-SULFAMETHOXAZOLE)

Effect:
Treatment of certain infections, especially urinary tract and middle ear.

Side Effects:
1) Nausea, indigestion.
2) Sulfa allergies such as skin rashes, blood-count disturbances.

Advice:
Never take for longer than recommended by your doctor.

BENADRYL* (DIPHENHYDRAMINE) See antihistamines.

BENZODIA ZEPINES

Effects:
1) So-called minor tranquilizers for chronic anxiety.
2) Induce sleep (sedation).

Side Effects:
Habit forming.

Advice:
Try not to take on a regular basis or you may not be able to do without them.

BRONDECON*

Effect:
Opens up bronchial passages; useful for treating asthma and emphysema.

Side Effect:
Palpitation, nervousness, upset stomach, nausea.

CATAPRES* (CLONIDINE)

Effects:
Same as Aldomet.

Side Effects:
Same as Aldomet (1) and (2).

Advice:
See Aldomet. Never stop this drug suddenly.

CHLORAMPHENICOL (CHLOROMYCETIN*)

Effect:
Antibiotic—effective against many bacteria.

Side Effect:
It may damage the bone marrow so that it can no longer make red blood cells, white blood cells, or platelets.

Advice:
May result in death from infection, internal bleeding, or severe anemia.

This drug, because of its danger, should be used only for certain serious infections such as typhoid fever and meningitis if you are allergic to penicillin.

CHLOROTHIAZIDE DIURETICS

Effects:

1) Increase in loss of water and salt from the kidneys; useful when there is accumulation of excess fluid in the body.
2) Lower blood pressure.

Side Effects:

1) Loss of too much fluid from the kidneys leading to weakness, dizziness, and thirst.
2) Loss of too much potassium leading to muscle weakness and abnormal heart rhythm.
3) Loss of too much sodium leading to lethargy and weakness.
4) Increase uric acid level in blood and occasionally precipitate an attack of gout.
5) Can raise blood sugar.

Advice:

Check with your doctor if you feel unusually weak or thirsty. Often, potassium chloride is prescribed with these pills. Do not stop potassium on your own while using water pills.

CHLOR-TRIMETON* (CHLORPHENIRAMINE) See antihistamines.

CIMETIDINE (TAGAMET*)

Effect:

Reduces stomach acid; used to treat peptic ulcers and esophagitis.

Side Effects:

Swelling of breasts.

CLINORIL* (SULINDAC) Similar to Motrin.

COGENTIN* See Artane.

COMPAZINE* (PROCHLORPERAZINE) See phenothiazine drugs. Used more often for vomiting.

CORTISONE DRUGS (STEROIDS)

Effects:

Reduces inflammation in tissues. Useful for certain

forms of arthritis, bowel inflammation, asthma, skin conditions.

Side Effects:

1) Raises blood sugar.
2) Thins bones; can cause spine collapse after long-term use.
3) Causes puffiness of face and shoulders.

COUMADIN* (WARFARIN SODIUM)

Effect:

Oral anticoagulant drug to be taken by people likely to have blood clots.

Side Effect:

Same as heparin.

Advice:

This medicine must be monitored regularly with a blood test called *prothrombin time*. The dose may have to be adjusted according to the result of the test. This test should be performed at least once every four to six weeks. Since many drugs can interact with Coumadin, never use any other pills without checking with your doctor first. Examples include phenobarbital or aspirin.

DALMANE* (FLURAZEPAM) See benzodiazepines.

DARVON* (PROPOXYPHENE)

Effect:

Pain reliever but does not relieve inflammation.

Side Effects:

Nausea, vomiting, dizziness.

DEXAMETHASONE (DECADRON*) See cortisone drugs.

DIABETIC AGENTS

Effects:

Release insulin and lower blood sugar.

Side Effects:

1) Hypoglycemia (low blood sugar).
2) Liver injury especially with Diabinase.
3) Allergy.

DIABINESE* (CHLORPROPAMIDE) See diabetic agents.

DIAMOX* (ACETAZOLAMIDE)

Effects:

A diuretic that is used primarily to reduce fluid buildup in eye in patients with glaucoma.

DIGOXIN
   Effects:
   1) Strengthens the heartbeat.
   2) Slows the heart rate.
   Side Effects:
   1) May cause nausea and vomiting.
   2) May cause abnormal heart rhythms, leading to pal-
       pitation or fainting.
   Advice:
   Check your pulse rate daily. If it falls below 60 per
   minute, or goes over 100 per minute, or becomes irregular, check with your doctor immediately.

DILANTIN* (PHENYTOIN)
   Effect:
   Treatment of seizure disorders. Occasionally used for
   side effects of Digitalis.
   Side Effects:
   Certain type of anemia.

DIURIL* (CHLOROTHIAZIDE) See chlorothiazide diuretics.

DONNATAL* See anticholinergics (contains phenobarbital,
hyoscyamine, and atropine).

ELAVIL* (AMITRIPTYLINE) See tricyclic antidepressant drugs.

ERYTHROMYCIN
   Effect:
   Antibiotic effective in most cases of pneumonia; good
   substitute for penicillin if you are allergic to latter.
   Side Effect:
   Nausea and vomiting.

ESTROGEN HORMONES
   Effect:
   Cause female characteristics. Used for control of menopausal symptoms and treatment of certain cancers such
   as breast or prostate.
   Side Effects:
   1) Fluid retention.
   2) Nausea.

FURADANTIN* (NITROFURANTOIN)
   Effect:
   Treatment of urinary tract infections.

Side Effects:

1) Nausea.
2) Lung inflammation causing shortness of breath.
3) Damage to nerves of hands and feet with numbness and weakness.
4) Inflammation of the liver.
5) Fever.

Advice:

Report any unusual weakness, trouble with breathing or feeling of numbness and tingling in extremities to your doctor.

FUROSEMIDE (LASIX*)

Effects:

Same as chlorothiazide, but more potent.

Side Effects:

1) Same as chlorothiazide.
2) Occasional hearing loss if administered in high doses by injection.

HALDOL* (HALOPERIDOL)

Effect:

Tranquilizer.

Side Effects:

Same as phenothiazines (1) and (2).

HEPARIN

Effects:

Prevents blood clots.

Side Effects:

Excessive bleeding from any area of the body.

HYDRALAZINE (APRESOLINE*)

Effects:

1) Lowers blood pressure by causing small blood vessels to open (vasodilatation).
2) Strengthens heartbeat.

Side Effects:

1) Blood pressure may fall too much when you stand up, resulting in dizziness or fainting.
2) Same as Pronestyl.

Advice:

Rise slowly to standing position after sitting or lying down.

HYDRODIURIL* (HYDROCHLOROTHIAZIDE) See chlorothiazide diuretics.

HYGROTON* (CHLORTHALIDONE) See chlorothiazide diuretics.

INDOMETHACIN (INDOCIN*)
Effect:
Relieves inflammation and pain in certain forms of arthritis.
Side Effects:
1) Stomach irritation and bleeding from the stomach.
2) Headache and dizziness.
3) Affects bone marrow.
Advice:
Same as aspirin.

ISORDIL* (ISOSORBIDE DINITRATE)
Effects:
A longer-acting form of nitroglycerin.
Side Effects:
Same as nitroglycerin.

KEFLEX* (CEPHALEXIN)
Effect:
Antibiotic effective in urinary and certain other infections.
Side Effect:
Same as penicillin.

LEVODOPA (LARODOPA*)
Effect:
Treatment of rigidity and tremors in Parkinson's disease.
Side Effects:
1) Nausea.
2) Jerking movements of head and neck.
3) Abnormal heart rhythms.
4) Lowers blood pressure.
Advice:
Use with caution in people with heart disease.

LIBRAX* See anticholinergics (contains Librium*).

LIBRIUM* (CHLORODIAZEPOXIDE) See benzodiazepines.

MELLARIL* (THIORIDAZINE) See phenothiazine drugs.

MOTRIN* (IBUPROFEN)
Effects:
Reduces joint pains and inflammation in certain forms
of arthritis.
Side Effects:
1) Nausea, indigestion.
2) Dizziness.
3) Rash.
Advice:
Use with caution in people with peptic ulcers.

NAPROSYN* (NAPROXEN) Similar to Motrin.

NITROGLYCERINE
Effects:
Opens up blood vessels and relaxes certain type of in-
ternal muscle as in the esophagus.
Side Effects:
Headache, flushing, dizziness.
Advice:
Tablets lose effectiveness after a time. Should be stored
in refrigerator.

NORPACE* (DISOPYRAMIDE PHOSPHATE)
Effects:
Same as quinidine.
Side Effects:
1) Nausea.
2) Urinary retention, mostly in men.
3) May cause weak heartbeat, leading to fluid accumulation in the lungs and shortness of breath.
Advice:
If you notice a decrease in urinary stream, see your
doctor.

ORINASE* (TOLBUTAMIDE) See diabetic agents.

OXACILLIN
Effect:
A modified penicillin that is effective against staphy-
lococcal infections.
Side Effect:
Same as penicillin.

PENICILLIN
   Effect:
      Antibiotic effective against most infections of the lungs
      and skin and meningitis.
   Side Effect:
      Allergic reactions, such as skin rashes, hives, and diffi-
      culty in breathing.
PERSANTINE* (DIPYRIDAMOLE)
   Effect:
      Opens blood vessels; reduces clotting by effect on plate-
      lets. Used now more frequently in treatment of po-
      tential strokes because of latter affect.
   Side Effect:
      Headache, dizziness.
PHENOTHIAZINE DRUGS
   Effect:
      Tranquilizers useful for chronic anxiety and psychotic
      behavior.
   Side Effects:
      1) Slurred speech.
      2) Stiffness of movement with tremors.
      3) Jaundice.
      All these effects disappear when the drug is stopped.
PHENYLBUTAZONE (BUTAZOLIDIN*)
   Effect:
      Relieves inflammation; useful for treatment of arthritis
      and bursitis.
   Side Effects:
      1) Stomach irritation and bleeding from the stomach.
      2) Occasional depression of bone marrow, leading to a
         decrease in red and white blood cells.
      3) Fluid retention.
   Advice:
      You should have a blood count before taking this medi-
      cine and should never take it for more than one week at
      a time.
PREDNISOLONE   See cortisone drugs.
PREDNISONE   See cortisone drugs.
PREMARIN* See estrogen hormones.

PRO-BANTHINE* (PROPANTHELINE) See anticholinergics.

PRONESTYL* (PROCAINAMIDE)

Effects:

Same as quinidine.

Side Effects:

Development of antibodies in the blood, leading to joint pains, pleurisy, weakness, muscle pains, and fever. These effects subside when the drug is stopped.

PROPRANOLOL (INDERAL*)

Effects:

1) Decreases work of the heart and thus relieves angina.
2) Slows heart rate.
3) Lowers blood pressure.
4) Prevents migraine headaches.

Side Effects:

1) May cause weak heartbeat, leading to fluid accumulation in the lungs and shortness of breath.
2) May cause asthma in susceptible people.
3) May lead to dizziness on standing up.
4) Abdominal cramps.

Advice:

Check pulse rate daily. If it suddenly falls below 60 beats per minute, check with your doctor immediately.

QUINIDINE

Effects:

Prevents abnormal rhythms and extra beats of the heart.

Side Effects:

1) Occasionally bleeding in the skin or other areas of the body may occur because of a decrease in blood platelets. This bleeding may appear as clusters of tiny, maroon spots on the skin.
2) Skin rashes.
3) Nausea, vomiting, diarrhea.

Advice:

If you notice purple marks on skin, see your doctor immediately.

STELAZINE* (TRIFLUOPERAZINE) See phenothiazine drugs.

SYNTHROID* (LEVOTHYROXINE)
Effect:
Treatment of deficiency of thyroid hormones.
Side Effects:
1) Nervousness.
2) Rapid heartbeat.
3) Sweating.
4) Increased bowel movements.
5) Weight loss.

TEDRAL*
Effect:
Same as Brondecon.
Side Effects:
Nervousness, palpitation, rapid heart rate.

TERBUTALINE (BRETHINE*)
Effect:
Opens up bronchial passages.
Side Effect:
Headaches, palpitation, nervousness, and cramps.

TETRACYCLINE
Effect:
Antibiotic—effective in urinary and other infections.
Side Effect:
Nausea and vomiting, diarrhea.

THORAZINE* (CHLORPROMAZINE) See phenothiazine drugs.

TOFRANIL* (IMIPRAMINE) See tricyclic antidepressant drugs.

TOLECTIN* (TOLMETIN SODIUM) Similar to Motrin.

TOLINASE* (TOLAZAMIDE) See diabetic agents.

TRIAMCINOLONE (ARISTOCORT*) See cortisone drugs.

TRIAMTERENE (DYRENIUM*)
Effects:
Same as Aldactone.
Side Effects:
1) Same as chlorothiazide (1).
2) Too much potassium retention leading to abnormal heart rhythm. This drug should be used only in combination with a chlorothiazide or furosemide.

TRICYCLIC ANTIDEPRESSANT DRUGS
   Effect:
      Relieve serious depression. Require several weeks of
      therapy before an effect is noticed.
   Side Effects:
      Serious and fatal abnormalities of rhythm of heart.
   Advice:
      These drugs should be used very cautiously by anyone
      with heart disease.

VALIUM* (DIAZEPAM) See benzodiazepines.

GLOSSARY OF MEDICAL TERMS

Absorption	Passage of dietary products and drugs from the gastrointestinal tract into the bloodstream.
Adrenal Glands	Endocrine glands sitting on top of the kidneys that produce cortisone, adrenaline, and other hormones that regulate fluid balance in the body and enable the body to respond to stress.
Anemia	A deficiency of red blood cells.
Anergy	Inability to mount an allergic response.
Aneurysm	Localized widening and stretching out of an artery.
Angina Pectoris	Chest pain that occurs usually on exertion when the heart does not receive enough oxygen. It disappears with rest within a few minutes.
Anorexia	Decreased appetite.
Antibody	Protein produced by lymphocytes in response to foreign material such as

bacteria, viruses, and bee venom entering the body.

Antigen — Foreign material that stimulates the formation of antibodies.

Anuria — Lack of urine flow.

Anus — External canal of rectum.

Aorta — Main artery of the body, coming from the left ventricle of the heart and branching into other arteries that go throughout the body.

Aortic Aneurysm — Aneurysm of the aorta.

Aortic Valve — Regulates flow of blood from left ventricle to aorta.

Aphasia — Difficulty in speaking due to damage to speech center of brain.

Arachnoid — Thin inner covering of the brain and spinal cord, lying beneath the dura.

Arrhythmia — Abnormal heart rhythm.

Arteriosclerosis — Hardening of the arteries leading to blockage of arteries and aneurysms.

Artery — Vessel carrying blood from the heart to the various organs of the body delivering oxygen and nutrients.

Arthralgia — Aches in joints.

Arthritis — Inflammation or damage to joints.

Atria — Small cavities of the heart that hold the blood before it enters the ventricles.

Auscultation — Listening with a stethoscope.

Bile — A suspension of fats and minerals delivered by the liver to the intestine through the bile duct. Aids in breaking down fat during digestion.

Bile Duct — A tube connecting the liver with the intestines.

Bilirubin — A pigment made in the liver.

Bradyarrhythmia — Abnormally slow heart rhythm.

Bradycardia — Slow heart rate.

Bronchi — Bronchial tubes that carry air between the windpipe and lungs.

Bulla	A large fluid-filled blister on skin.
Bursa	Fluid-filled sac overlooking joints.
Capillaries	Tiny, thin blood vessels that receive blood from all arteries. They deliver oxygen and nutrition to the cells of the body and pick up waste products.
Carcinoma	Type of malignant tumor of an internal organ or skin.
Carpal bones	Wrist bones.
Cerebral Hemorrhage	A stroke caused by a bleeding blood vessel in the brain.
Cerebral Thrombosis	A stroke caused by blockage of an artery going to the brain.
Cerebrovascular Accident	Stroke.
Cervical area	Neck area.
Cholecystitis	Inflammation of the gall bladder.
Cholelithiasis	Gallstones in the gall bladder.
Clavicle	Collarbone.
Colon	Large intestine or bowels. Situated between small intestine and rectum, it carries waste products to rectum.
Congestive Heart Failure	Poor heart function leading to accumulation of fluid throughout the body and decreased circulation to the major organs of the body.
Conjunctiva	Membrane covering whites of eyes and inner eyelids.
Constipation	Abnormally infrequent bowel movements, usually formed and hard.
Coronary Insufficiency	Heart pain due to lack of oxygen that lasts for more than thirty minutes.
Coryza	Nasal stuffiness.
Cyanosis	A blue color under the fingernails and/or the lips due to low oxygen concentration in the blood or poor circulation.
Cystitis	Inflammation of urinary bladder.
Diaphragm	Tentlike muscle that separates chest from abdomen and helps to inflate

the lungs during inhalation of air.

Diarrhea — Abnormally frequent bowel movements, usually loose and unformed.

Diastole — Period between heartbeat when heart is relaxing.

Digestion — The process of breaking down food into smaller compounds in the gastrointestinal tract. Carbohydrates are broken down to glucose, proteins to amino acids, and fats to fatty acids.

Diplopia — Double vision.

Diuretic — Water pill; causes excess urination and loss of salt in urine.

Diverticulum — Small narrow outpouching of an area of the gastrointestinal tract. Usually occurs in large intestine (colon).

Duodenum — First part of small intestine and most susceptible to peptic ulcer.

Dura — Tough outer covering of the brain and spinal cord.

Dysarthria — Difficulty in speaking.

Dysphagia — Difficulty in swallowing.

Dyspnea — Shortness of breath.

Dysuria — Pain on urinating.

Ecchymosis — Red-purple blotches under skin due to bleeding.

Edema — Abnormal accumulation of fluid anywhere in the body.

Ejaculation — Ejection of semen.

Embolus — A piece of blood clot that breaks off from its original place and travels through the bloodstream to another area.

Endocrine Gland — Gland that produces hormones.

Enzymes — Chemicals that regulate body functions. Every cell makes enzymes for itself. In addition, organs such as the pancreas make enzymes that work in other areas of the body.

Epididymis — Small gland lying on testes.

Epigastrium	Midline part of the abdomen just below rib cage.
Epistaxis	Nose bleed.
Eructation	Passing gas through mouth.
Erythema	Redness.
Esophagus	Muscular tube carrying food from throat to stomach.
Flatus	Gas passed by rectum.
Focal Seizure	Convulsion limited to part of the body.
Frequency	Urinating more often than normal.
Gall Bladder	A sac connected by tubes to both the liver and the intestines; stores extra bile made by the liver.
Gland	An organ that makes chemicals to perform specific functions in the body.
Grand Mal Seizure	Generalized convulsion with loss of consciousness.
Heart Murmur	A noise made as blood travels through the heart. Usually occurs as blood goes past a heart valve.
Heart Valve	Valves that open and close to regulate flow of blood through the chambers of the heart.
Hematemesis	Vomiting of blood.
Hematoma	A collection of blood.
Hematuria	Blood in urine.
Hemiparesis	Weakness of arm and leg on one side of the body.
Hemiplegia	Paralysis of arm and leg on one side of the body.
Hemoglobin	The compound inside red blood cells that carries oxygen.
Hemoptysis	Coughing up blood.
Hepatic	Referring to liver.
Hiatus Hernia	Protrusion of a portion of the stomach into the chest through an opening in the diaphragm.
Hormone	A chemical made in one area of the

	body that travels through the bloodstream to do its work in another area.
Hyperglycemia	Abnormally high blood-sugar level.
Hypertension	High blood pressure.
Hypoglycemia	Abnormally low blood-sugar level.
Hypotension	Low blood pressure.
Hypothalamus	An area of the brain that lies near the pituitary gland and regulates emotions, appetite, sleep patterns, thirst, and the pituitary gland.
Hypoxia	A deficiency of oxygen.
Icterus	Jaundice.
Impotence	Inability to have an erection.
Incontinence	Inability to control flow of urine or stool.
Inguinal area	Groin.
Intermittent Claudication	Pain in the legs on walking caused by lack of oxygen in the leg muscles.
Jaundice	A yellow color in the eyes and skin due to accumulation of a pigment called bilirubin in the blood.
Laryngitis	Inflammation of larynx.
Larynx	Part of throat encompassing voice box and vocal cords.
Left Ventricle	Strong pumping chamber whose role is to pump blood rich in oxygen through the arteries to the cells of the body.
Lumbar puncture	Spinal tap.
Lymphocytes	Cells produced in the lymph nodes of the body that produce antibodies.
Lymphoma	Tumor of lymph nodes.
Malabsorption	Inability to absorb food properly from the intestines, usually leading to diarrhea and weight loss.
Mandible	Jawbone.
Melena	Black bowel movement due to blood in stool.
Meninges	Lining of the brain and spinal cord.

Meningitis	Infection of the lining of the brain and spinal cord.
Metacarpal bones	Hand bones.
Metastasis	Spread of tumor from its site of origin.
Metatarsal bones	Bones of the foot.
Mitral Valve	Regulates flow of blood from left atrium to left ventricle.
Monoplegia	Paralysis of one limb.
Myalgia	Aches in muscles.
Myocardial Infarction	Heart attack in which a piece of heart muscle dies from lack of oxygen.
Myopia	Nearsightedness.
Myositis	Inflammation of muscles.
Neoplasm	Tumor.
Nephritis	Disease of the kidneys.
Nocturia	Awakening at night to urinate.
Obstipation	Lack of passage of stool or gas through rectum.
Oliguria	Small, inadequate volume of urine.
Orthopnea	Shortness of breath when lying down on the back.
Orthostatic Hypotension	A blood pressure that falls to a low level when one arises from a lying or sitting position.
Otitis	Inflammation of ear.
Palpation	Examination by feeling.
Pancreas	Organ lying on top of the spine in the upper abdomen that provides enzymes for digestion of food and insulin for regulation of blood-sugar levels.
Papule	A small firm excrescence on skin.
Paraplegia	Paralysis of both legs.
Paresthesia	Sensation of numbness and tingling or pins and needles.
Paroxysmal Nocturnal Dyspnea	Shortness of breath that awakens you from sleep.
Peptic Ulcer	A hole in the lining of stomach or

	small intestine due usually to too much acid production by the stomach.
Percussion	Examination by gently rapping one finger on another and noting quality of sound.
Peristalsis	Squeezing action of the intestine.
Peritoneum	Tough lining of the abdominal cavity.
Peritonitis	Inflammation of peritoneum.
Pharyngitis	Inflammation of pharynx.
Pharynx	Throat.
Pituitary Gland	Major endocrine gland of the body, located at the base of the brain.
Platelets	Blood cells that prevent excessive bleeding by forming clots at the site of injuries.
Podagra	Painful swelling of ball of foot around big toe.
Polycythemia	Too many red blood cells.
Polydipsia	Increased thirst.
Polyphagia	Increased appetite.
Post-Ictal State	Temporary state of unconsciousness after a seizure.
Presbyopic	Difficulty in vision associated with aging.
Psychomotor Seizure	Abnormal behavior caused by a convulsion.
Pulmonary Artery	Artery that carries blood to the lungs to receive oxygen.
Pulmonary Edema	Accumulation of fluid in the lungs, usually because the heart is functioning poorly.
Pulmonary Embolus	An embolus to an artery in the lungs, usually from a vein in a leg.
Pulmonary Valve	Regulates flow of blood from right ventricle to pulmonary artery.
Pulmonary Vein	Vein that carries blood rich in oxygen from the lungs to the left atrium.
Purpura	Purple blotches under skin due to bleeding.

Rales	Crackling sounds heard in chest through a stethoscope, usually indicating inflammation or fluid in air sacs.
Red Blood Cells	Blood cells that carry oxygen to the cells of the body.
Renal Lithiasis	Kidney stones.
Right Ventricle	The heart chamber that pumps blood through the pulmonary artery to the lungs to receive oxygen.
Sacrum	Small of back.
Sclera	Tough outer layer of eyeball; white of eyes.
Scrotum	Sac containing testes.
Sedative	Drug that induces sleep.
Seizure	Convulsion. Abnormal, uncontrollable, movements of body.
Small Intestines	Bowel between stomach and colon where most of digestion and absorption of food takes place.
Spleen	Internal organ located in the upper left side of abdomen responsible for removing old red blood cells and fighting infection.
Sternum	Breastbone.
Strabismus	Deviation of eyes from normal, symmetrical alignment, "cross eyed."
Stroke	Sudden damage to the brain, usually leading to paralysis and often impairment of speech and thinking.
Subarachnoid	Under the arachnoid.
Subdural	Under the dura.
Supraclavicular	Lying above clavicle.
Syncope	Fainting episode. Short, transient episode of unconsciousness.
Systole	Contracting of heart.
Tachyarrhythmia	Abnormally rapid heart rhythm.
Tachycardia	Rapid heart rate.
Tarsal bones	Ankle bones.
Tenesmus	Discomforting sensation of incom-

	plete evacuation of stool.
Thorax	Chest cage.
Thrombophlebitis	Abnormal blood clot in a vein.
Thrombus	Abnormal blood clot clogging an artery or vein.
Thyroid Gland	Endocrine gland lying over the windpipe in the lower neck. Makes a hormone called thyroxine that regulates the body's metabolism.
Tinnitus	Ringing in ears.
Trachea	Windpipe connecting mouth and nose with bronchial tubes.
Tranquilizer	Drug that calms an individual.
Tricuspid Valve	Regulates flow of blood from right atrium to right ventricle.
Urethritis	Inflammation of urethra, the canal leading out of urinary bladder.
Vein	Blood vessel that brings blood from the capillaries back to the heart.
Ventricles	Main pumping chambers of the heart.
Vertigo	Dizziness characterized by spinning sensation.
Vesicle	A small fluid-filled blister on skin.
White Blood Cells (Leukocytes)	Blood cells that fight infection by killing bacteria and viruses.

INDEX

C

D

E

Quality PLUME Books for Your Reference

☐ **NATURAL COOKING: THE *PREVENTION*® WAY edited by Charles Gerras.** A guide to good cooking and good eating that offers more than 800 health-filled recipes from *Prevention*® magazine. It shows how meals rich in nutritional value can be prepared without sugar, salt, or deep-fat frying.
(#Z5260—$5.95)

☐ **THE TAPPAN CREATIVE COOKBOOK FOR MICROWAVE OVENS AND RANGES by Sylvia Schur.** From breakfast for one to dinner for twenty—prepare over 400 delectable dishes designed for microwave ovens or standard stoves.
(#Z5146—$3.95)

☐ **THE SUPERMARKET HANDBOOK: Access to Whole Foods by Nikki and David Goldbeck.** This book will prove invaluable to any shopper concerned with the quality and nutritive value of foods available in today's supermarkets. It will help you to understand labels and select foods with a discerning eye, and provides easy, low-cost ways of preparing and using whole foods in place of processed foods. "An enormously useful and heartening work!"—*The New York Times* (#Z5151—$4.95)

☐ **THE WORLD ALMANAC® WHOLE HEALTH GUIDE by David Hendin.** Based on over six years of extensive research, this valuable guide offers information on such topics as finding and checking out a doctor, patient's rights, saving money on prescriptions, mental health problems, child abuse, the elderly, and sources for acquiring even more information.
(#Z5145—$4.95)

☐ **THE ORIGINAL BOSTON COOKING-SCHOOL COOK BOOK, 1896 by Fannie Merritt Farmer.** A facsimile of the first edition of *The Boston Cooking-School Book.* Includes more than 1,300 recipes as well as illustrations, glossary, and index.
(#Z5167—$4.95)

☐ **AMERICAN FOLK MEDICINE by Clarence Meyer.** An alphabetical listing of virtually every ill the flesh is heir to—with fine, time-tested home remedies that use herbs, garden vegetables, fruits, and other natural ingredients.
(#Z5097—$3.95)

In Canada, please add $1.00 to the price of each book.

To order these titles, please use coupon
on the last page of this book.

Quality PLUME Guides of Special Interest